The Dilemmas of Brief Psychotherapy

The Dilemmas of Brief Psychotherapy

James P. Gustafson
University of Wisconsin–Madison
Madison, Wisconsin

Springer Science+Business Media, LLC

Library of Congress Cataloging-in-Publication Data

On file

Grateful acknowledgement is made to quote from the following sources:

T. F. H. Allen and T. B. Starr, *Hierarchy: Perspectives for Ecological Complexity*. Chicago: University of Chicago Press, 1982. Reprinted by permission.

Carol Bly, *Letters from the Country*, copyright 1973, 1975, 1978, 1979, 1981, by Carol Bly. Reprinted by permission of HarperCollins Publishers.

J. B. Calhoun, ed., *Environment and Population*; reprinted by permission of Greenwood Publishing Group, Inc., Westport, CT. Copyright ©1989 by Praeger Publishers.

Joseph Campbell, *Masks of God: Occidental Mythology*. Copyright 1964 by Joseph Campbell. Used by permission of Viking Penguin, a division of Penguin Books USA.

E. Canetti, *Crowds and Power*. New York: Continuum Publishing Group, 1972. Reprinted by permission.

Antoine de Saint-Exupery, *Wind, Sand and Stars*, copyright 1939 by Antoine de Saint-Exupery and renewed by Lewis Galantiere; reprinted by permission of Harcourt, Brace & Company.

Ted Hughes, *Shakespeare and the Goddess of Complete Being*. Copyright 1992 by Ted Hughes and reprinted by permission of Farrar, Strauss, and Giroux, Inc.

Thomas Merton, *Seven Storey Mountain*, copyright 1948 by Harcourt, Brace & Company and renewed 1976 by the Trustees of the Merton Legacy Trust; reprinted by permission of the publisher.

K. Koryani, Morbidity and rates of undiagnosed physical illnesses in a psychiatry clinic population. *Archives of General Psychiatry*, 36: 441–449. Copyright 1979 American Medical Association.

Phyllis Rose, *Parallel Lives*. New York, Random House, 1981. Reprinted by permission.

ISBN 978-1-4613-5744-5 ISBN 978-1-4615-1837-2 (eBook)
DOI 10.1007/978-1-4615-1837-2

Originally published by Plenum Press, New York in 1995
Softcover reprint of the hardcover 1st edition 1995

10 9 8 7 6 5 4 3 2 1

To my parents, Jane and the late Paul Gustafson
To my wife, Ruth
And to my children, Ian, Caitlin and Karin

Preface

The question of brief psychotherapy is whether it can be more than shallow. I believe it can go deeply, in most cases, even in a single hour, to what I call the patient's dilemma. This is why psychotherapists and students come to watch me work, and why they will want to study this book. It is my reply to *The Complex Secret of Brief Psychotherapy* (Gustafson, 1986), which I wrote ten years ago, when I asked how the intrapsychic, interpersonal, and systemic perspectives fit together.

I have been helped to write this book principally by three readers and friends, Ruth Gustafson, Michael Moran, and Peter Miller, with some additional help from Lowell Cooper, Mike Wood, Vance Wilson, and Myron Sharaf. My students in the Brief Psychotherapy Clinic of 1993–1994 contributed lively discussions on the first fourteen chapters. They include William Ayetey, Shirley Dawson, Suzy Freedman, Tamar Kelson, Donna Kiley, Maureen Leahy, Sara Long, Deborah Lynn, Michael Maze, Karin Ringler, and Steve Sutherland. I am indebted to Dee Jones, for her skills in typing the manuscript with wonderful accuracy, speed, and organization.

I also want to credit Ryle (1990, 1994) for his prior use of the term *dilemma* in psychotherapy, which was known principally in England until his recent publication. Comparison of his use and my use of the term, I believe, will show that he uses it in a restrictive and pathological and cognitive sense to mean "false choices and narrow options (p. 99, 1994)," while I mean something of more structural and general importance in the life of man as a group animal. I have discussed this further in *Brief Versus Long Psychotherapy in Practice* (1995, especially Chapter 18).

Finally, I want to thank all my patients, who have taught me everything I need to know by showing me my errors, and all my far-flung students in workshops who have also seen the holes in my accounts and pointed them out to me. I am very glad for the Door County Summer Institute, in particular, where I have taught week-long workshops on brief psychotherapy the last two summers in one of the most beautiful settings in the country. I conduct workshops all over the country, and sometimes the world, but it is very pleasant to have a home base, where students of this extraordinary subject may come to visit me.

[illegible]

... in a more ... [illegible] ... together ... [illegible] ... "OQ." ... While I ... something ... [illegible] ... and ... importance in the life of ... a group ... [illegible] ... in *Brief ... Psychotherapy in Practice* ... [illegible] ... Chapter ... [illegible]

Finally, I want to thank all my patients, who have taught me everything I need to know by showing me ... and all my ... students in workshops who have also seen the ... in the ... and ... them to me. I am ... for the ... Summer ... in particular, where I have taught week-long workshops on brief psychotherapy the last two summers in one of the most beautiful settings in the country. I conduct workshops all over the country, and sometimes the world, but it is very pleasant to have ... home base, where students ... ary subject may come to visit me.

Contents

Introduction

Nothing is harder to find than an honest portrait of misfortune.
WEIL, 1940

SELECTIVE INATTENTION

How are we to be useful in the patient's current episode of distress, briefly, with the twelve or six or two sessions allotted, *and* yet borrow from the fertility of the unconscious? To meet the challenge of any case in an hour, we have to see first what the patient is looking for, consciously. Yet, he always overlooks what will stop him from finding it. Thus, he is always unconscious of what is most important.

The Case of the Missing Lion

For example, a patient complains of hair-pulling and consciously wants to stop. Behavioral ideas from her therapist help her combat the urge, but the urges cannot be resisted after the brief therapy concludes and she is separated from her helpful doctor. I am consulted. Here is the usual situation where a behavioral, cognitive, psychodynamic, or strategic idea has assisted the conscious aim to some extent, yet the unconscious remains a force to be reckoned with. It will be her undoing unless we can put our finger on what it is up to. The design of the unconscious will be left out of the conscious story of the patient, and, very often, that of the therapist; there will be big holes in the account.

It turns out that this young lady is a perfectionist in nursing, whose perfect plans cannot help but tighten her up. As long as she has to be perfect, she is going to be anxiously aware of her flaws. This is the first hole in the story: if she cannot ease her aims, she is going to need *some* way to unwind—such as pulling out her lashes. This is a hole on the outside surface of the story, generated by the way she tries to fit herself into the working world.

There is another hole, as in all cases, on the inside surface of her shadow self.

She has a dream fragment of "a murderer in the family!" This turns out to refer to the crude man who will become her father-in-law when she gets married in a few months. Despite her plans for a perfectly orderly life, she is marrying into a family far from perfect. She is roiled and rattled by her outrage at this impending situation.

This patient consciously looks for an end to her pulling out of lashes, and gets assistance from a conscious plan of psychotherapy; yet, she and the therapist overlook the two big holes where the unconscious will undo their work.

My method of methods is to accept whatever method the patient has for getting where she wants to go, and whatever method the therapist has for furthering this conscious aim, and to bring into focus what both of them overlook. I think that this selective inattention (Sullivan, 1954, 1956) is what keeps brief psychotherapy from being effective. If the patient and therapist overlook the holes, they cannot repair them.

AFTER THE EPISODE OF BRIEF PSYCHOTHERAPY

There is a great tendency in the field of brief psychotherapy to conclude the story—after resolving an episode like this one of the nurse getting anxious and pulling out her lashes—as if one lived happily ever after. This is a myth, or a machine for the suppression of the drift in time (Levi-Strauss in Charbonnier, 1969). Actually, living happily ever after without further disturbance would mean becoming fixed. A fixed person dries up, repeating himself. This is sterility.

In actual time, the only reliable way to be refreshed is to allow oneself to become disturbed by the unfamiliar. Such a life of individuation goes from one episode of difficulty to another and thus the self becomes larger rather than smaller. It takes on more of being, over time.

Thus, the way of individuation is a succession of episodes, like the episode of brief psychotherapy, whose terms change over time. Sometimes the individual can manage the new episode himself; sometimes he can extend the education gotten from an episode in brief psychotherapy; sometimes he needs a succession of episodes in psychotherapy, either the continuity of long-term therapy or a return for a second or third brief therapy or consultation.

Generally, the episode that brings the patient to brief psychotherapy is a dilemma that has two horns. The outer horn is where the patient is being hooked by the world, like my nursing student hooked on being perfect and thus becoming tense. The inner horn is the force from the unconscious that is too much to handle, like my patient becoming roiled and rattled by injustice. If she passes through the horns of this dilemma, of having a difficult semester and marrying into a family with injustice, her dilemma is apt to be ongoing.

She remains a character bent on perfection. Thus she is apt to get hooked on new occasions for performing. She remains a character whose shadow side is still fiercely aroused by injustice. So she is apt to get hooked on new occasions of injustice.

Therefore, I always conclude an episode of brief psychotherapy by posing the possible shapes of the ongoing dilemma, hoping to help the patient keep her eyes open for the next struggle. I work to make her selective inattention less for what is surely coming.

PSYCHIC INFLATION, DEFLATION, AND VACILLATION

The most reliable way for a patient or any individual to keep from getting stuck is to continue his own education, both outward about how the world works, and inward about the unconscious. Both are great subjects. Gaps in education can be very costly.

For example, a patient complained to me about lack of sexual interest in her husband. This puzzled her, for she liked to think of him physically when she was away from him. But when he turned from his sports television network to touch her, she laughed and hurt his feelings. She did not understand why she reacted as she did. She did know it was thrilling to meet new men when she traveled. Even to flirt a little got her going more than performing sex with her husband.

I replied that she only half understood the Eros. She knew that Eros thrived on being new, but she was still amazed that the old and daily routines with her husband left her unwilling to respond except with laughter. Is it possible, said she, to be excited about someone you have lived with for twenty years?

I said, yes, it is, but only if he is new himself, and if you are new yourself, by continual rebirth. Then the two of you meet anew. Otherwise, lovemaking is going to become tedious. Thus, becoming fixed has great consequences, and an education about how this works can point the way to release.

Another patient showed the reverse problem. She knew that living coldly with her husband was barren. She tried to come alive with another man full of poetry. This was very fine, but it threw her into a panic when the poetic man hesitated to go on. She fell into the abyss of her childhood, which was abandonment and attack by her cruel father, for taking this step toward coming alive.

Lack of education about how the outer world, and the inner world, work can be disastrous. Thus, I believe that we psychotherapists need to know about resolving the dilemma of an episode in brief psychotherapy, but we also need to know what it takes for continuous, ongoing development.

Thus, this book is also about the back-and-forth of the spirit, between the outer world and the inner world, which is a fertile life. Any less knowledge and we fail our patients at some point. In this precise sense of knowledge of the path of the spirit, this is a religious book.

Jung mapped a great deal of this subject. He showed how the narrow focus of the conscious mind is naturally compensated by the dream focus of the unconscious mind. He also showed how the dream focus is apt to be carried away by what he called *psychic inflation.* The only recourse is to come back to outer reality and its *psychic deflation.* This back-and-forth between conscious and unconscious perspectives is not an elective exercise for those with nothing better to do. It is a matter of life and death.

As Campbell points out in his extraordinary introduction to *The Hero with a Thousand Faces* (1949), it is extremely dangerous to be *disoriented* about the spirit. To be captured by a stultifying situation is to become dispirited, like Anna Karenina (Tolstoy, 1875–1877) in her marriage to Karenin and in their circle of society. This is psychic deflation, where the spirit is punctured like an inner tube, and the breath or pneuma leaves. This is bad, but it is even worse to become puffed up in the psychic inflation of Anna's love for Vronsky, which defies all the limitations of society. It is going to be hauled down and dismembered.

Thus, balance between the two dangers of living dispiritedly and being puffed up in romanticism is of the greatest importance. However, many balance themselves by lack of commitment, fearing to be big or small, merely oscillating between the two conceptions.

We as psychotherapists are asked nowadays to show that our patients have a "medically necessary" condition to justify payment for treatment by a third-party insurer or HMO. In my opinion, psychic deflation or inflation or vacillation are medically necessary conditions *if* the patient grasps the psychic disaster and is prepared to work at it. If he grasps his psychic failure, he is sure to be anxious and depressed. He will be particularly distressed about some needed adjustment in his life concerning love or work. In this precise sense of the *Diagnostic and Statistical Manual of Mental Disorders,* Fourth edition (DSM-IV), he will have an adjustment disorder, 309.28, with anxious and depressed mood. Of course, he may have worse complications, as anxiety and depression drive him into such things as the affective and psychotic disorders of Axis I and the rigidities of Axis II.

THE FOCUS NEEDS TO BE DOUBLE: THE DILEMMA

The trouble with any learning about the three propensities of psychic deflation, inflation, and vacillation is that bringing one region of the psyche into focus always puts another region into shadow. Thus, Jung helped us enormously by putting dreams into focus, yet his weakness was to know too little about the machinery of the external world.

How are we to learn anything about our subject by bringing it into focus, without losing something extremely important in shadow? After all, the entire subject of brief psychotherapy is about choosing a focus and sticking to it for solving an episode in the patient's life. Indeed, the nature of focus is to privilege a single area and neglect other areas. It is like the acute vision that we get from the fovea of the retina: excellent in what it can do, but dangerous unless compensated by peripheral vision.

Ten years ago, while writing my first book of brief psychotherapy (Gustafson, 1986), I posed this very problem to the field. How could we so acutely focus on the psychodynamic inner world without losing focus on the dangerous outer world? How could we so acutely focus on the systemic outer world without losing focus on the inner world? How could we so acutely focus on the interpersonal world without losing focus on both the inner world of dreams and the outer world of systemic hierarchies?

It appeared that focal brief psychotherapy was operating with one eye, and only with the fovea. Each school had its own fovea. Now this is perfectly understandable. Each school is based on a premise, or *lemma,* about what is valuable to do in psychotherapy. It is always one thing. The group's agreement about the object of scrutiny is what holds the group together.

When I wrote my first book, I knew all three kinds of lenses—inner, transitional, and outer—were extremely important. I could do no more than say so, and show the power of Freud and Reich on the inner world; Sullivan, Alexander and French, Winnicott, and Balint interpersonally; and Selvini-Palazzoli, Bateson, and Maturana on the outer world, and so forth. It has taken me another ten years to figure out how these three regions can be drawn together in a relatively simple way.

My reply at last is that the focus I take for psychotherapy is the patient's dilemma. Invariably, instead of the usual one thing, this puts into focus two things, as William James (1902/1958) called for (Gustafson, 1967), that is, the patient's conscious focus and his unconscious shadow or periphery. This makes psychotherapy like any skilled art or sport, where, for example, the piano requires attention to the right hand until the musician can half forget it and attend to the left hand. The two together are the music.

THE THREE PARTS OF THIS BOOK

The right hand in psychotherapy is attunement to the patient's conscious intention. It is tantamount to the skill in locating what he is looking for in any hour of work. My students like to call it empathy, or feeling-with. The left hand in psychotherapy brings into focus what is overlooked because of the conscious focus. Part I of this book is about achieving this double focus on dilemma in the beginning, middle, and end of brief psychotherapy.

The trouble with clarity of focus about the relatively simple dilemmas is that there are only four kinds of them: subservience, delay, overpowering, and basically faulted. Because they map most of the territory we will encounter in brief psychotherapy, we are apt to lose stories that are more complex. In a more complex story, the two-part harmony of melody (conscious) and accompaniment (unconscious) breaks into the polyphony of many voices. In Part II, we get the simple, two-part, variations down first, before tackling complex compositions.

The trouble with facility about stories is that we can get so readily between conscious and unconscious mind that we do not dwell long enough in contemplation of either the outer or the inner world. In Part III, we take this upon ourselves with the analysis of dreams, and with the analysis of the coming social world. Finally, we conclude with a small series of follow-up studies that illustrate the importance of inner strength, outer places to land, and an accurate map for the journey.

THE READERSHIP

Allow me to suggest only one more idea in concluding this introduction, which concerns the readership of this book. I spent the year of 1993–1994 in my Brief Psychotherapy Clinic alternating between consultations with the patients of third- and fourth-year residents and psychology fellows in the clinic, and discussions of their reading of the chapters of this book. It is quite obvious to us all that third- and fourth-year residents are fully able to use the focus of dilemma in a very practical way in their work. It is also quite obvious that the first-year residents can use the concept with great clarity from the very outset in our seminar on "The Dilemmas of Managing with Dangerous Personalities," and that the second-year residents can do the same in my section of "Contemporary Models of Psychotherapy." A brief introductory course on brief therapy could make good use of the book in one semester.

Indeed, taxi drivers understand the idea, and aunts, and patients coming for first visits. The word "dilemma" is used intuitively by most adults, adolescents, and even children. I am not recommending using the word, although some will take me to mean this concretely. I mean that the concept is readily available, but always peripheral and used only on occasion. Persons and patients and doctors know what it is but do not understand its profound significance in their lives.

What I am trying to say is that it is not a high idea, which needs to be saved for the elect of psychotherapy. It is a very down-to-earth idea and it has two horns that will make themselves felt with great hurt. However, it turns out that getting through the horns of a single dilemma in brief psychotherapy can set the individual on a road of a long series of dilemmas that ascend through all of Creation. I believe that sophisticated readers will find enough for them on this journey. The low leads to the high as we have always known, yet it leads there only for those who have an adequate map or guide. This book could be seen to have two plateaus, from the common plateau of clinical work in brief psychotherapy in Chapters 1–9, to the perspective of more complex individuation in Chapters 10–15. We begin in hell on the horns of the Devil Himself!

Part I

Beginning, Middle, and Ending Dilemmas

In a poem, one line may hide another line,
As at a crossing, one train may hide another train.
KOCH, 1993

It turns out to be a paired universe, of left and right, up and down, outer and inner, extensors and flexors, striated muscle and smooth muscle, sympathetic nerves and cholinergic nerves. Perhaps we map the universe this way because our bodies are constructed of these opposites. In any event, if we get only one half of the equation we lose our balance and tip over. In the metaphor of Koch's poem, we get by the first train, only to be struck by the second we weren't looking for!

Therefore, the opening part of the book is about readiness for both trains, in beginning, middle, and end. Most of my students do better with the first train than with the shadow, or second train. Usually, they have not been taught about its coming. As Sullivan would say, the patient always leaves out the most important part of the story, and it is our expertise to know what to look for.

In other words, I pose the three acts of the drama of brief psychotherapy as pairs of problems, or dilemmas. Dilemmas have two horns, upon which we can be impaled if we are not watchful. I suppose we were once more likely to be run through by wild boars, while now the trains have a greater shot at us.

Act I is the opening situation of first interviews, in which the patient hopes to get somewhere and the doctor to make an adequate appraisal of what it would take to get there. The first problem is how to ride the hope, which is refreshing. Too often it is neglected by the doctor anxious to ask enough questions so he is not misled. This is Chapter 1. The second problem of first interviews, following hard upon the first problem, is to reckon the hazards of the journey in advance. Too often this is neglected by the doctor anxious to believe in the patient's readiness to undergo trial and tribulation. This is Chapter 2.

Act II is the middle situation, which is often called working through. Usually, this is the weakest, most amorphous or cloudy part of books on psychotherapy. I propose that it has a very decided structure, the structure of the patient's dilemma, with its two horns, its two slopes, and its two catastrophes. I illustrate the classical female dilemmas in Chapter 3, and the classical male dilemmas in Chapter 4. Of course, nowadays, men and women often have both kinds.

Act III is the ending situation, usually called by the word termination, which is grim by its association with dying and euphemistic by its association with terminals. The first problem is to conclude a difficult episode with a patient by getting him or her through the valley of the shadow of death, like divorce, or firing, or illness. This gives a tight ending, after which the patient is anxious to resume the great American virtue of self-reliance. This is Chapter 5. The second problem is that dilemmas do not go away just because a particular episode has been concluded or even solved. Some patients are comfortable with facing the ongoing nature of the dilemma of their lives, that is, that it will return in many new episodes. They like a loose ending, so the therapist can be found again, like a good mentor, or general practitioner. This is Chapter 6.

Acts I, II, and III of the drama of brief psychotherapy follow the same logic as the monomyth (Campbell, 1949), which is the common plot of all myths of the hero the world around. Probably, it is the universal route of renewal for man and woman stuck in degenerating situations. Act I is the departure to an alternative world. Act II is the discovery of something valuable to live for. Act III is the reentry with this discovery and preparation to defend it. Of course, this same sequence is tragic if the discovery is overwhelming and cannot be faced without destruction.

Every night and day has this cycle as well, as we depart our daytime conscious mind for dreaming at night and return in the morning to insert the dream in the regime of daily life (see Chapter 13 for discussion of this daily rejuvenation that we can free up in brief psychotherapy). This is our royal road, if we can only find how to use it. It is the sonata form of music.

For me, every single hour has this full cycle of departure, discovery, and return. I find what the patient is looking for, what he overlooks (and finds with my help), and what is his dilemma in owning it and going on. Even a tragic finding can sometimes be borne as a dilemma whose pain is shared (Winnicott, 1971b, Chapter 18; Gustafson, 1986, Chapter 7). In this sense of the single hour, I propose a method that is timeless and time bound (John Strezlec, personal communication). The cycle of the available sessions also follows the same logic. If I proceed through Acts I, II, and III in the first hour, I repeat this in all the subsequent hours as if each were the first (Winnicott, 1971b; Gustafson, 1986, Chapter 7). Nevertheless, the beginning hours determine if departure from being stuck is plausible, the middle hours are full of discovery of the patient's dilemma, and the concluding hours test the patient's ability to defend his discovery going away from me.

Chapter 1

The Freshness of First Sessions

She was looking for what she calls "characteristic moments." "That's when people actually take control of their interview . . ."
ANNA DEVEARE SMITH, QUOTED BY BERNARD WEINRAUB, 1993

First meetings have a great potential if we know how to bring it out. Winnicott (1971b) certainly knew, from his work with children:

> I was struck by the frequency with which the children had dreamed of me the night before attending . . . here I was, as I discovered to my amusement, fitting in with a preconceived notion. . . . Either this sacred moment is used or it is wasted. (pp. 4–5)

Adults in trouble often resemble children, for they too want to give themselves away. (Of course, some adults, and children, dread trusting anyone and become more inaccessible the more they are troubled. We will discuss this in Chapter 2.) Yet we must know how to conduct ourselves to allow them this unburdening. Even if we are persuaded by Winnicott's picture of help, we will need to be careful about several technical points. In our own anxiety, we can get in the way. Often, these interviews get off on the wrong foot.

WHO IS LOOKING FOR SOMETHING

The Docile Body

Second-year residents in a clinic have to file the best report they can for the clinic chart from the first session. Thus, they are impelled to take control of the interview, which leaves the patient in the role of the one controlled by questions. The style is gentler than in a courtroom, but the patient ends up in the predicament of a witness against himself, that is, in Foucault's (1975) phrase, as a docile body, or as a not so docile body barely able to contain himself. The residents get a half hour, and then it's my turn.

I begin by summarizing what I have heard, but I reverse emphasis, from what the resident has found out, to what the patient, or the person who sent the patient, was looking for from us!

The Case of a Woman Looking for a Doctor to Give Her Lithium

A middle-aged mother of three had begun by telling the resident that she had lost her old doctor who had given her lithium, and now sought a new one as a replacement. The resident felt obliged to find out all she could about what had gone so far wrong that the patient needed this serious drug. She fired a volley of questions to pin down the disturbance, and instead pinned down the patient far behind the baseline, where the patient played very weakly, and began to twitch and look appealingly at me.

All I did was to reverse the field, *by saying simply that she was looking for* a doctor to give her lithium, which seemed to be very important to her. Oh yes, she said, it was terrible when she was twelve and depressed, and mother ignored her, even while her brother turning blue from asthma got rushed to emergency rooms right and left. Then at sixteen she became manic, which forced mother's hand, yet the doctor attributed to adolescence the fact that she could not study at all with her racing thoughts.

I responded (now that the patient had taken over the interview) that she had been let down too many times. Oh yes, she said, and it is happening right now, because this very brother is living with her and terrorizing her in his drunkenness with plots to trap the skunks under the house with bear traps! She has nightmares of her children falling into them, but again her mother tells her she worries too much, and she is again woefully ignored. She tells me she is relieved by our talk, because I am on her side.

So the resident gets her evidence for the report in the clinic chart, but it is evidence driving straight at us on the strong wind of the patient's passion for an ally, rather than evidence fleeing from us under covers.

Problem-Posing

This is precisely the difference between what you get when the patient is the active subject versus what you get when the patient is the passive object. I am not against questions per se, such as are necessary about disturbances that are dissociated and about symptoms that could be signs of physical illness. The order is the thing. A patient who has told her story can later bear some inquiry without losing her dignity. I follow David Malan's (1979) example in this, which I remember vividly from my visits with him at the Tavistock Clinic. He brought out the subject in the first half of the interview, whereupon he wheeled like a naval officer and took two paces back to survey the damages objectively.

Yes, the great problem of the first meeting is to establish the subject in her own story. It is quite like the problem of Brazil's Minister of Education in the liberal Goulart government, Paulo Freire (1970), who was called on to teach millions of illiterate peasants how to read and write Portugese. When he sent teams of smart city people out to the country to instruct the peasants, nothing happened. When these smart city people reversed themselves by showing pictures to the peasants of the peasants' own world and asking them what words seemed fitting to them, the peasants could not stop talking, reading, and writing. The first approach is what Freire called the Director Culture, which reduced the peasants to a culture of silence. The second approach is what Freire called problem-posing, which brought out the full subjectivity of the peasants in their own generative language. We are in danger of being a Director Culture, and putting our patients in a culture of silence. This is why I pose pictures of what the patient is looking for.

The Patient Has Been Sent by Someone Else

Yet it is a mistake to assume the patient is looking for something, unless we make sure that someone else has not been looking for something by sending us the patient! The patient has been in such a muddle that she has driven some other helper crazy. So the helper is looking for somebody else to do something, and that is the only line to such an interview that will make any sense. The patient is only delivering a message, and will not come to life in Freire's sense of generativity unless we bring out the presence of the message-sender that stands behind the play.

Getting a patient like this is like picking up a tangled ball of yarn (Gustafson, 1986; Selvini-Palazzoli, 1985). The more you pull on it, the worse it can become. Usually, several referring parties have already tried this, and given up in frustration. So it is not a good idea to dive into the yarn and tug on it with a hundred questions. A much better idea is to find the loose end. The loose end turns out to be in the mind of the person who sent the patient!

A Case of Whirliness

When the patient's chart comes in a wheelbarrow, you can look for the start of a very unsatisfying exercise. A seventy-year-old married mother of five was preceded by her voluminous records, which included three different cancers, cardiovascular disease including stroke and high blood pressure, depression, anxiety, headaches, dizziness, hot flashes, paresthesia, and so forth. She herself was as garrulous as her chart was long. Not only did she have an endless list of complaints, but she also had quite a list of enthusiasms. Obviously, the lady had a lot of energy, and was too much for anyone to manage.

The resident made a game effort to wrestle with all of this. She certainly wrote a lot of it down. After a half-hour, both she and the patient were very tense, for so much was wrong. This problem saturation (White and Epston, 1990) is a very unpleasant state. But how was the mess to be sorted out in the quarter of an hour left to me? Certainly, there was a great deal of organic illness, and very likely there was a great deal of psychological overlay. For example, her complaint of "whirliness" in her ears was so idiosyncratic that I felt quite sure it would lead to her peculiar world. Still, I also felt I would be as lost as the resident and the patient if I grabbed hold of "whirliness" and ended up in a dust devil myself.

Instead, I backed away from all the details and asked the lady *how she got to us?* It seemed that she was sent by her oldest daughter, who had told her that the doctors were missing something. What had given the daughter that impression, I asked. Well, the old lady was especially worried about her husband. He had always been too trusting in the family business, and now that he was so dizzy with Ménière's disease, he was leaving it in very bad hands. It made her so mad! She felt absolutely helpless!

At last, the patient, the resident, and I felt some relief, for the patient was getting some catharsis and calm. She went on to say that her daughter didn't like to hear this distress about her own father, and her friends didn't like to hear about it either, so there was really no one to tell. She had to listen to her husband, but no one wanted to listen to her!

What did her husband complain about most, I asked. "Whirliness," she replied. I smiled to myself, for I saw that whirliness had been passed from the old man to his wife, quite as the ill fathers had passed on their physical complaints to their wives and daughters, who had felt stuck taking care of them in the 1890s in Vienna. In other words, we had run into the phenomenon discussed by Breuer and Freud (1895/1966) in their *Studies on Hysteria*.

In hysterical patients, whirliness or some other physical complaint is *acquired* when the patient is in a helpless rage like this lady was. She has fastened on to the very complaint that gets her husband taken care of. This is what is called suggestibility. Now, she too will be taken care of. Similarly, the hysterical patients on Charcot's ward got epileptic "seizures" when he introduced epileptic patients who were of dramatic interest to himself and his colleagues (Havens, personal communication).

As Sullivan (1956) showed, hysteria is a very simple operation. It begins when the patient imitates a malady she has witnessed. Hysteria only becomes complicated by the number of imitations attempted by the patient. Once the patient has got the talent, she can even invent illnesses without seeing them in others, simply by attending to the multifarious body sensations aroused by anxiety. In general, a single imitation of an illness, like the odor of burnt pudding in Lucy, the fainting spell in Katherina, or the sensory loss on the leg of Fraulein Elisabeth, indicates a more benign case that can be resolved in brief psychotherapy, while the large collection of imitations of illness, like in Frau Emmy and Anna O., indicates a more malignant case that will not be resolved in brief psychotherapy (Breuer and Freud, 1895/1966). Now, I could simply say to the patient that coping with her husband was too much, and she needed occasionally to talk with someone about it besides her daughter. She

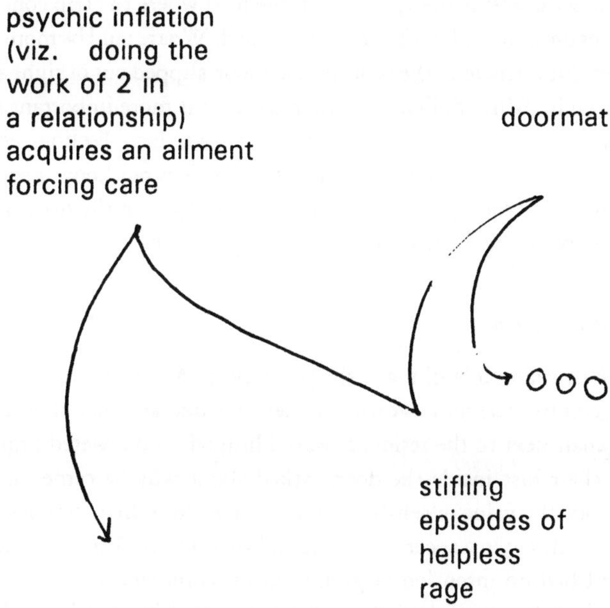

Figure 1.1. The horns of the devil in hysteria, a rampant dilemma.

agreed and left happily, but perhaps the greatest relief will be that of the daughter, the message-sender, because we took in her message.

WHAT IS THE GAP IN THE STORY

Sullivan's Hypothesis

So if the first problem of the interview is to establish what is being looked for, by the patient or his sender, the second problem is to reckon what it will take to reach the desired destination. Almost always, the patient is doing something to take himself off the track.

This self-defeating something will be left neatly out of his narrative (not consciously). The patient is himself unaware of his own part in derailing himself. This is what Sullivan (1956) called selective inattention:

> And the selective inattention is so suave that we are not warned that we have not heard the most important thing in the story—that it has just been dropped out . . . so that we just do not notice the gap where it belongs. (p. 52)
>
> Selective inattention is the classic means by which we do not profit from experience. (p. 50)

Sullivan rightly notes that selective inattention is of "profound theoretical significance" (p. 48), because it is the very turn in the road where the trip continues or gets derailed. It goes unnoticed. It will not be mentioned. What could be more important to psychotherapy? Nevertheless, the concept itself soon slipped out of sight after Sullivan put his finger on it. Why? Sullivan's answer is that it is more important to feel secure than to know what's going on. Thus, the concept was lost. Feeling secure helps an individual to keep his standing in groups, even if he does not know what he is doing.

Therefore, my second problem is to listen for the gap in the story. I will look for the patient to veer away from it, whenever we get close.

A Case of Intimidation

An extreme example will make the point clear. A wiry middle-aged man came in warily, in combat fatigues, wearing something like an Australian bush hat. He declined the chair next to the resident, waved him off, and lowered himself carefully into another chair just inside the door. Asked about why he came in, he began to pontificate about the value of self-help organizations for schizophrenics like himself. Occasionally, he threw in a sneer at doctors and their rotten drugs. Obviously, he was in charge, and had no intention of giving up his command.

The resident was tactful, and the patient settled in. We learned little more, because the resident was pinned down by his own politeness. He was half right, for without this concession, the patient would break off in a second. The problem was that the resident did not know how to keep one foot still while letting the other foot circle toward the disturbance like a compass. Instead, he got in occasional queries that the patient dismissed readily. Finally, as time ran out, the resident became a little desperate and jumped on the subject of the patient's mother, which had rattled the patient when run by him earlier. The patient exploded into curses and fled the room.

Thus, you often dare not go straight for the gap in the story. If you do, the results are apt to be exciting but unworkable. You have to back away from the gap and move toward it gradually, with a logic the patient can follow. For example, this patient could have been offered a smooth transition (Gustafson, 1986; Sullivan, 1956) as follows: "Obviously, you have gained a great deal from self-help organizations. Let's go back to when it was working best." The implication is clear. There has been a falling off, which we will have to reckon with if we are to be of any help. We will first establish the patient's success. This relieves the patient of his dread that we wish to unsaddle him: not at all. It has already happened, and we only want to help him get back on top where he is comfortable.

In other words, the doctor has a dilemma. If he lets the patient stay on top in grandiose control, the doctor will not get near the disturbance. If he takes the patient off his high horse, he will have a patient who is helpless on foot and explodes out of the room like this man did. The most probable way through the horns of this dilemma is to establish the patient's success more firmly by history, and then note that it is something *in the world* that unsaddled him. Thus, I will say: "You were

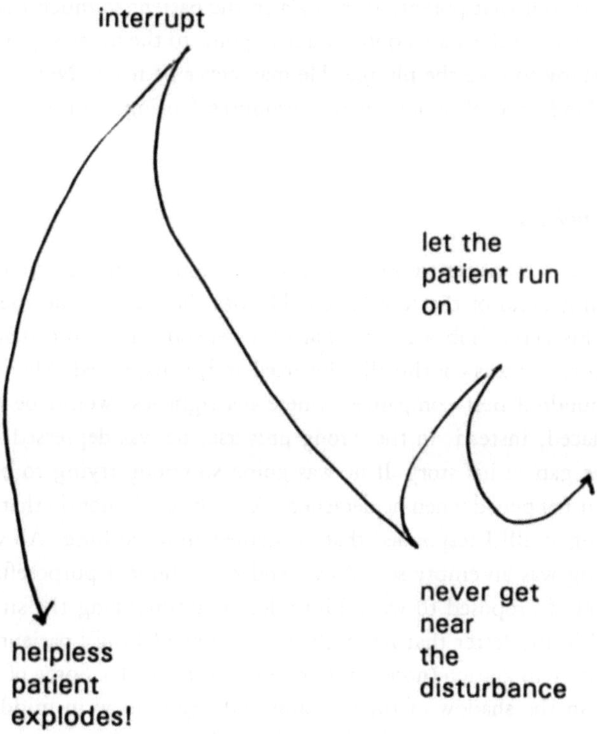

Figure 1.2. The doctor's dilemma with the manic patient.

doing so well in your organization for self-help, until something went wrong. Otherwise, you would not have landed in the hospital." This will be a lot easier for the patient to take, for the world did it to him, not the doctor. Still, highly manic patients will not allow you to do even this, for they have to be charging around continuously to overlook their helplessness.

Sullivan's Romance

Now while it is true that a skillful interviewer can discern the gap in the story and move into it with tact, it is by no means true that the patient will be able to work with this decisive turn in the road. Sullivan (1956) made the job sound workable, when often it is not at all:

> Thus we try to proceed along the general lines of getting some notion of what stands in the way of successful living for the person, quite certain that if we can clear away the obstacles, everything else will take care of itself. . . . The patients took care of that, once I had done the necessary brush-clearing. (pp. 238–239)

Uncovering is just not that potent. It may alarm the patient so much that he clings like a drowning man to the status quo. You may point to the necessary crossing, but he may not be ready to take the plunge. He may never be ready. Notice that I have shifted from a landscape of action, which promises footing, to a seascape, which arouses terror.

A Case of Napoleon

This man was a manager whose hero was Napoleon, in the very precise sense of the autocrat and general of the Revolution. He was there to set the country right. Unfortunately, his actual job was less that of a general, and more that of a chief steward. Therefore, he was continually thwarted and, thus, vexed. He wished to be in one of the hundred best companies, where his rightness would be recognized. Since he was placed, instead, in the wrong universe, he was depressed.

I posed the gap in his story. If he was going so wrong trying to be on top of everything, what happened when he detached? Well, he could not do that. He would end up not caring at all! I responded that he seemed all or nothing. All was ruining him, and nothing was an empty sea. As we ended the hour, I purposefully did not conclude. Rather, I proposed to write him a letter summarizing the situation.

I proposed in my letter that he might be like one of Jung's patients who were captains of industry in Zurich (note, captains and not generals). Some of them could find a new self in the shadow of their dreams and begin anew in middle age, and some could not. Like any other medical consultant, I proposed more tests, and in his case, a test of his ability to bring dreams.

He brought a number, and then desisted. He stuck to his guns at work, buttressed by the resident giving him antidepressant and antianxiety agents. Thus, he kept his favored footing, and declined a passage at sea. (In a letter from the patient responding to this account, he gives a slightly different picture. In his dreams, he is more of a Western cowboy than a Napoleon and in danger of going off by himself into the sunset like in the movies. This alarms him, and drives him back toward his familiar stewardship of the company. So, he tends to be overresponsible in his persona, or throwing off all responsibility in his shadow. A middle ground or third position is a very slow development in such cases (see Gustafson, 1995, especially Chapter 11 on Jekyll/Hyde).

WHAT COMPANY IS NEEDED

Winnicott's Dream Dive

It is not necessary to pose the sea passage in shadow in the form of dreams. There are other tests of readiness or nerve. For example, patients who are being trampled can be told that they are probably not up to facing certain difficult people, or certain feelings like anger, or certain assignments to show their skill.

But like Winnicott, I like to propose a dive into a dream, once the drift of the present course is charted. Dream analysis has several advantages. One is that it drops us into the feelings that must be borne to get across the sea. A second is that it provides a precise and individual map of the terrors of the sea in the particular patient. His unconscious has already X-rayed the gap. We are testing the readiness of the patient to face his own X-ray. A third is that we will discover if there is satisfaction for the patient in the descent, which will buoy him through further arduous passages.

A Case of a Black Hole

A forty-year-old divorced mother of two came for a first appointment after her sixteen-year-old daughter elected to leave her to go live with the father. Her distress was evident. The resident linked the patient's distress to the patient's own childhood. She felt burdened as a teenager by her own mother's confiding distress, and wanted to go to her father for refuge. Her father hadn't wanted her. Thus, she had gotten sexually active with a boy, to find comfort that she could not get from her father. Now her daughter wanted to get away from her, and go to the father, where the daughter could get away with being sexually active because she would not be so closely watched.

Thus, the resident had done a very nice job of linking the pain of the present to the pain of the past. In my turn, I just stayed with the pain, because the patient could bear it without the grave complications of suicidality and psychosis and because the resident had room to take the patient. How had she lost custody of this daughter, I asked.

Her husband had been abusive and mean to her. She had felt helpless, but then began to feel like taking it out on her girls. She confessed this to the Family Court, whereupon the court decided that both parents were injurious to the girls, and awarded joint custody. This was altogether too much for her to take, for opening her mouth had gotten her kicked in the teeth. She felt altogether swindled, since her husband had been literally brutal, while she had only felt like it and asked for help *not* to become that way. She felt like screaming in the court, "Those children are my life," but instead collapsed in shock.

Like many who have become victims, she had been too open and too trusting. She had mistaken Family Court as help, rather than as a contest for possession of her girls. By staying with her pain, we had gotten a most vivid picture of her posture of trust that allowed her participation in her own tragedy.

I asked her for a recent dream. She gave me a long and powerful, or epic, dream that culminated in a scene in her childhood bathroom: There was a white picket fence around a black hole in the floor, with a little four-legged black chair over the hole. The white picket fence took her to her American dream of a family, while the black chair and hole seemed to draw her from potty training into it as if it were an immense gravitational field. She became extremely anxious, and tried to wake up, and imagined her boyfriend was standing by her bed. This last image was a hypnagogic illusion, but terribly important because it showed her how her need threw her into the arms of someone she hardly knew.

The reader may ask what has been gained from the individual map of the dream that we did not already know from our map of her stance of excessive trust. First, we get a vivid picture of her American dream: she loves white picket fences so much, so to speak, that she is not apt to look closely at who is living inside them. Second, we get a vivid picture of her terror, which reaches back into the early childhood of potty training: if the light is still dim so far back, there is still ample suggestion she had reason to fear her parents early in her life. Third, we see that her terror literally drives her into her excess of trust: she leaps out of what is most dire into the arms of what is most idealized.

Her helpers now knew about more than her excessive trust. They also knew something of its motives, namely, that she is like a poor, overrun country trying to defend itself from one enemy by opening its doors to another enemy because it so desperately requires protection. This idealization of the second enemy, while understandable, is exceedingly dangerous to her. This will become a crucial subject of subsequent discussions.

I think the dream was also directly relieving to the patient, for it provided a vehicle in which we could travel with her from what is most beautiful to her, to what is most terrifying, to the jump to illusive safety. The dream itself had been bewildering, but the retelling to us slowed it down, gave her company—that is, pause and comfort, and allowed her to take it in as a set of signposts to heed. Patients are often like frantic travelers until a guide can settle them down so that they can use the maps they carry unwittingly inside themselves.

Chapter 2

Perils at the Outset

The . . . [doctor] . . . during this period may be compared to a traveler standing on top a hill overlooking the country through which he is about to journey.
ALEXANDER AND FRENCH, 1946, P. 109

THE FIRST SLOPE

In the first session, riding the longing of the patient is only sensible if it is balanced by a sharp outlook for dangerous turns. The first look will be ahead for a drift or a fall from the present position. Where will the slope of the patient's fall take him?

Perhaps the danger cannot be contained in the outpatient clinic. The patient may go right through the floor, and end up in peril. If lucky, he will end up in some asylum like an inpatient service, or jail, or a detoxification center, before destroying himself or someone else, or both.

So it is imperative that we do our very best to imagine the patient going from bad to worse, and get prepared. The best way I know to become fully mindful of the limitations of outpatient help is to go to the inpatient service for a week and see what comes in from the outside world.

A Week on the Inpatient Service

All of the people in inpatient service are in unbearable pain. They vary in how they respond. The lessons here are repetitive, but essential, like the circles of hell in Dante's *Inferno.*

Suicide: A Case of a Young Man with a Death Car

Some are near the quitting edge of life. Actually, all of the patients here are in despair, but some are actually prepared to dispatch themselves. For example, one young man came to the hospital in what I called his death car. He had it full of all his earthly possessions and rigged up with a tube for gassing himself, like a burial mound for a warrior on wheels. It sat ready in the parking lot of the hospital for a country ride to eternity. How are we to know when we can let him go? Eventually we must.

Unfortunately, I find most of our residents replying to this critical question with a point of few that I call digital. The entire point of view is standard and taught by the faculty. That is, they regard patients as either suicidal or not suicidal. Often, they ask the patient if he is or he isn't. If he isn't, then he can go. If he is, then he has to sign a contract stipulating that he will not harm himself.

The absurdity of this digital map is that the patient may not be suicidal ensconced in his room on the ward away from the injuring world, while he becomes profoundly suicidal as soon as we seem not to care by letting him pass through the front door. This is why I prefer an analog map of the territory of despair. It presupposes that the suicidality of the patient will vary wildly with the territory. So I do not ask *if* he is or isn't, but *where* he is and *where* he isn't. This entire book is a set of field theories, as in physics (Kaku, 1994).

Most patients in despair are kept going by one of two things: by believing their fortunes will improve, or by somebody else wanting them to stay around (Havens, 1965, 1967). Our young man with the death car had neither. By his late twenties, he no longer believed he could hold a job, and he no longer believed that his family wanted him around as such a loser.

So we supplied the caring that he lacked by refusing to let him go. He asked to go. He said he was no longer suicidal. I reckoned that the method was at hand, the prospects hopeless, and the love gone. Therefore, I refused, and he, relieved, agreed with my appraisal. In several weeks, he rallied assiduously with family and friends, and responded to a plan for retraining so that we could entrust him to the world again.

This is the big thing. We must read the patient's despair for his prospects and for his connections, objectively, because he can mislead us, subjectively. The latter will fluctuate with the territory. The slower forms of suicide, like alcoholism and drug abuse, sexual promiscuity, gambling, and the life of the ailment in borderline personalities, have a similar terrain, and oblige us to pose similar questions. Where is control? Where is it lost? What is there to live for and with whom?

Finally, there is one sense in which the idea of a rational contract is decisive. Because control is a matter of place, the patient can be given responsibility for getting himself to safety before the grip is gone. Thus, we needed to say to the young man with the death car, once improved, that we lacked the godlike powers to foresee when some new setback between outpatient sessions would be more than he could bear and we would not be there to get him to safety. Only he could do that. Only if he could bear that responsibility could the resident be his doctor (Kernberg *et al.*, 1988). He felt he could. Indeed, he was relieved to be given an important job.

Homicide: A Case of Murdering the Doctor

If homicide is rarer than suicide, it still must be looked for in every suicidal display as its shadow. Assume the patient would like to take someone down with him. Ask not *whether* he is revengeful, but *how close* he has come to the deed, and *where* and *when* and *how?*

I had the gruesome opportunity to consult with an English hospital over the murder-suicide of one of their registrars (a resident is called a registrar in England) by one of their patients, where the lack of reading the shadow was obvious in retrospect.

The patient was a thirty-year-old paranoid schizophrenic from Scotland, who had had an acute psychotic break in his late teens. Thereafter, he never worked. Instead, he drifted around the north for about ten years. At thirty, he showed up in the south at this hospital complaining that his life was ruined, that he was the victim of a plot in his grammar school, and that the drugs he was given in Scotland made him worse.

The registrar was ambitious and decided he could get this patient going. I never did learn what it was about this patient that incited such optimism in his doctor, because the principals did not live to tell the story, and because the chart says so little. Suffice it to say that they met weekly for about three months in what was called intensive psychotherapy. The patient was moved to get a job, in which he lasted a week. He quit, complaining of people being against him. From here, it was all downhill for a year until the terrible end.

The registrar now came to his senses a little, and saw that the patient could not cope without antipsychotics. He insisted; the patient resisted. At about this time, records came from Scotland. Ominously, they recorded two arrests for assaulting neighbors who were noisy. The patient had nearly strangled two different offenders, but somehow desisted from finishing his murderous work.

The registrar was scared enough to back off at this point. His idea was to defuse the clash by diffusing the contact into visits every several months. The patient did not become less intense. Having had his romantic hopes aroused for a career, he now felt the backing off as a betrayal by the registrar. Several months later, the registrar began to get bizarre love letters in his mailbox daily. The patient was wooing, madly.

The registrar finally asked for help. The consultant agreed that the situation had become desperate, and proposed that the patient be transferred to a center where a team of mental health workers would look after him. The registrar told the patient of this decision over the telephone. The next day, after hours, the patient came in, caught the registrar in the hall, and asked for a few words privately. Once the door was shut, the patient murdered the registrar and then himself with a revolver.

The consultant had been right that this patient needed a team to take care of him so that he would not fix so forcefully on a helper in isolation. The terrible trouble was that he had already fastened. Like the wife who is finally freeing herself of a violent husband, the registrar was in greatest danger shutting the door.

Very strict counsel against convening with this patient might have saved the registrar's life. Sounder yet, the powers of the hospital could have met with this patient to tell him of the transfer, instead of leaving it to the isolated doctor. Having to face the hierarchy of the hospital might have given the patient pause in his revenge. These are, of course, late measures, which do not always work, as we read in the newspapers, where judges, attorneys, post office colleagues, but mostly wives and children, are murdered for having aroused hope that could not be fulfilled.

Psychosis: A Case of a Call from Elvis Presley

The third great problem that cannot always be managed in the outpatient clinic is psychosis, even when it poses little threat of violence to self or others. More than half of the patients on the inpatient service just cannot take care of themselves in their dilapidated states of mind and body. Some are senile old folks, some chronic schizophrenics, some manics, some involutional, some in psychotic depressions, and some are having first breakdowns.

Interestingly, they all turn out to have problems of residence (Beels, 1992). These patients are marginal people who go to pieces when they lose their boardinghouse, that is, their school, their family, or their group home. A decent boardinghouse is a precious niche, because it affords little responsibility to interact, yet some possibilities to ward off alienation. It protects, therefore, against the great terrors of intrusion and abandonment.

Take this protection away and a psychosis takes its place as a kind of delusional alternative, a refuge in madness. A patient dreamt very precisely of this security, in his case with his mother, as two beautiful teeth connected by a thin silver wire. When he lost her, the connection was severed, and he went promptly into a manic psychosis (Jacobson, 1953). This is the kind of sudden disaster that occurs so often at graduation from high school, or college, or even graduate school. The alma mater has been a good enough boardinghouse, and then the patient is shoved out the door.

Often, the protection erodes in a slower and less conspicuous way. For example, a young man from Glasgow got up very early to work as a milkman, spent the day with his girlfriend, and played in a rock and roll band at night. Since he could not stay awake twenty-four hours a day, something was going to go, and, naturally, it was showing up for the milk route before dawn. He got fired, whereupon his girlfriend dropped him for lack of money. He was so downhearted that he could no longer play in the rock band, so he lost his last tie and went mad. His psychosis began with a call on the telephone from Elvis Presley in America, inviting him to come over and become a rock star (Gustafson, 1967).

Once these patients begin the career of psychosis, it may be very difficult to get them out of what Michael White (1989) has called the "in-the-corner lifestyle."

They settle there, in the security, of sorts, of a low-level boardinghouse. (The dynamics of obsessive–compulsive disorder are similar. I will discuss them in Chapter 11.) White and his colleagues have had some remarkable success challenging some of these people about their careers so that they jump to a higher level. Some, of course, do not move an inch, and some have a so-called unique outcome and then go to pieces.

Returning from the inpatient to the outpatient service, we take with us a sharp eye for the three great perils in the drift of the patient's present life: suicide, homicide, and psychosis. Whether it is one, two, or all three of these calamities that is looming, we need to face the worst that is possible. The patient will leave it out. It is up to us to extrapolate from what the patient does tell us to the very darkest hour or to the most terrifying second. The relevant questions include: How close did you come? What held you back? What was strangest about this moment or this hour? What is most embarrassing to tell about this?

Often, I find it better to make statements, while leaving plenty of room to be corrected. I assume that it is worse than they can say, unless I say it first. So I will hazard statements like: I imagine you *did* lose control. When you are in a temper, you become a *different* person. As with drinkers, double what the patient admits to and you will often be closer to the truth. As with drinkers, bring relatives and friends and helpers into the room, and you will also be apt to be closer to the truth.

Finally, I find it crucial to assume that the dire situation will return under certain conditions. I need to think over what will bring back these conditions. I need also to consider *at what point* the patient still has a chance of getting himself to help, and when he is too far gone. So, my alliance with him is good only up to a certain level of disturbance. I had better know that, or I will expect too much of our rational agreements.

THE SECOND SLOPE IN SHADOW

If You Think This Is Bad

It is hard to watch patients slide downhill; we like to think we can put them on a gentler slope. But often the alternatives are worse. I have learned about all of these by missing them. So little had been written to warn me of misplaced optimism. An exception is David Malan's cautionary tales (1976a, 1976b, 1979).

It turns out that these tales fall into a few types, like Aesop's Fables. First, there are the patients who have a place only if they are officially sick. This is a vast army of those with chronic pain, depression, agoraphobia, obsessive–compulsive disorder, hypochondria, neurasthenia, and so forth, who have qualified thereby for a pension. A rule of thumb is that they are not about to give up their pension and end up with nothing, but I am willing to be proven wrong by a determined individual. So to the executive who has ended up flat on his back after folding in two different corporations I say that most men I know will never risk a third disaster. He in particular probably ought not to try, since he is so unknowledgeable about defending himself. This way of posing the problem has the virtue of testing his resolve, and of posing the actual danger on the slope that is in shadow.

Second, there is the vast army of lonely people, whose lives become grayer by the day. They wanly appeal to us to help them find company. Only there are always powerful reasons why company is not a good idea. Usually, it is because they are taken advantage of by just about anyone who can reach them. So they are actually out of danger, if miserable, via distance. Often, they get some connection from work, because it is impersonal (Guntrip, 1968). While they complain that this is too little contact, they are almost never prepared to take risks to get closer. They are usually right to forgo closeness.

Third, there is the vast army of persons who are underachievers. They do not finish theses, or they drop out of college after a year, or they can't bring themselves to fix their houses, and so on. Usually, they have a sinecure to fall back on, such as their guilty parents, who take them in, or their indulgent spouses, and so forth. Usually, they lack work habits. When they also lack drive, grit, and resilience, how are they ever to compete for scarce jobs with people who do have all of these formidable qualities? Indeed, they cannot, but, again, I am willing to be proven wrong by a particular individual.

The officially sick, the lonely, and the underemployed have in common that they complain of marginality, yet are not about to get in the flow. They may surprise us, but it is judicious for us to assume that the flow is too dangerous. At least, it is well to take a very good look before we recommend they get in the water.

Sometimes it is very difficult to see into this history because it has been put away for being too disturbing. It is dissociated, which is to say it is in a compartment of the mind for which there is little or no access, even for the patient himself. I attempt to reach these places routinely, in the latter half of the first interview, by asking for the hardest periods in the patient's life. I try to get a feel for them, and I try to find out what acts were performed when the patient was most disturbed, and finally how the patient got through them at all.

Very disturbing periods will be left out, when the patient himself has had to get rid of them by dissociation. When I am trying to find my way around in this kind of dark, I will ask for the three earliest memories as a kind of projection test (Mayman and Faris, 1960) for deeper hints.

The Case of a Woman Sleeping with a Knife under Her Mattress

A thirty-year-old woman with post-partum depression came to me preoccupied with fear about herself and her family dying. The resident and I were somewhat alarmed by what she said she did when in the grip of fear: After leaving her parents for college, she would barricade her door at night in the dormitory and sleep with a knife in between her mattresses. Obviously, she had her reasons to get ready for assault. It was unclear what prompted her.

Getting nowhere in that murk, I threw the light in a different direction by asking her in an off-hand manner for her three earliest memories. I guessed they would be more unguarded. Her first was of biting on a shoe. The feeling of this memory took her to being hurt by criticism from her grandmother. Her second memory was of her mother ironing. The feeling of this took her to feeling extremely bored, while her mother was very busy. Her third memory was of playing with a neighbor boy, who was run over by his parents as he and she played in the driveway. The feeling of this was of terror of dying or of being blamed.

She slipped directly from this third, frightful scene into her rage at her sister, who tormented her but whose actions were ignored by the parents. In desperation, she had attacked her sister with a knife. Thus, we reached the mystery of how she had become a bearer of knives. The good news was that she could feel similar rage at her husband without violence and without being rejected by him.

This is the kind of abyss that Balint (1968) called "the basic fault." In this place, the child is unprotected. It concerns a history of gross intrusion and abandonment, such as we find when parents are cruel, incestuous, desperate, mad, drunk, or just plain cold. In a thirty-year prospective study of over six hundred children, about a third underwent this disaster of childhood (Werner, 1989). Two-thirds of these children's parents defaulted so grossly that the children never achieved anything but marginality. One-third got away to neighbors, teachers, or relatives and made it through surprisingly well.

These latter children have circumvented destruction by finding someone to be with them and to be like (Gustafson, 1986; Reich, 1949), lifting them out of the abyss of the basic faulted childhood, which now lays in shadow, an extremely dangerous slope they dread getting near again, as in "A Case of a Woman Sleeping with a Knife under Her Mattress." This is also true of adults who have been shattered in experiences like the Vietnam War. These people need to stay on top of things by making themselves marginal, yet they may also look in from the outside and contemplate getting back in the flow. Some can with company, and some get worse for the attempt. This first group have benign basic faults, and the second malignant basic faults (Balint, 1968).

Noble Causes

Often, a patient who is sliding away into the margins will propose to us a way of saving himself that is impossible but attractive as a kind of noble cause. We are invited into collusion. If we accept, we will be blamed later, with great bitterness, for not getting him to his ideal.

A little list of such projects may give a sense of them as a class. A thirty-year-old man who had quit four attempts at psychotherapy proposed a fifth, if he could have a therapist who was like a friend he once had in college who took him hiking and showed him the great beauty of nature. A fifty-year-old man who had devoted his life to his daughters, like a kind of Pere Goriot (Balzac, 1835/1946), proposed that he needed my help to rescue one of them who had gone astray. A forty-year-old man who had conducted a holy war against his bureaucratic superiors, like a kind of Ralph Nader, proposed that I should help him win this war, even though he was one against a hundred and increasingly exhausted.

A woman who was fired ten times as a saleslady for sheer neglect of her accounts took to bed reading murder mysteries, waiting for a therapist who would get her motivated. A woman who had borne ten children and who could not have an eleventh for medical reasons proposed that she have a break from all her labor and have her patriarchal husband take her place at home. A man who had devoted his entire life to saving an alcoholic beauty collapsed when she committed suicide and wanted himself to be saved by a like effort, despite ruining himself by continuous drinking, eating, and ignoring his work.

I am not suggesting that we just turn these people down flat. I am saying that we have to propose that there is a double cusp to the catastrophe (Sashin, 1985). The slope they are going down is the first cusp. The noble slope that is shadowy and that they propose for themselves is the second.

A Case of a Patriot Who Had to Be in the Army

A twenty-five-year-old, single young man wishing to join R.O.T.C. came to us asking for a letter stating that he was well. The only problem was that he had been hospitalized several times after strange and violent episodes that made no apparent sense and that led to a diagnosis of schizophrenia.

With us, he was very friendly, entirely coherent, and absolutely clear in a complete examination of his mental status. The only odd thing about him was that he studied the ceiling during most of the interview. Asked about this, he claimed to be interested, from his work, in heating systems.

His medical chart, including an inpatient discharge summary, told us little, and confirmed that the diagnosis of schizophrenia had been made by several competent doctors in our department. The patient felt this was a mistake, that antipsychotic drugs were bad for him, and that he had done very well without the diagnosis or the drugs for half a year.

Furthermore, he was very fervent about wanting to give something back to his country by military service. He had just started graduate school again. He begged us to help him.

We were in a difficult dilemma. If we agreed with the previous doctors, he would feel unfairly crushed. If we agreed with him, we might be colluding with a

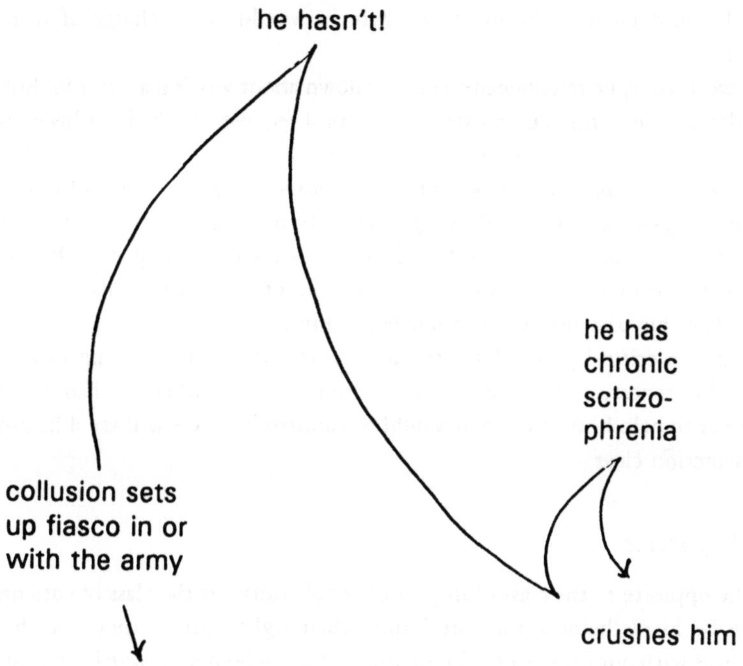

Figure 2.1. The classic dilemma with the chronic mental patient: from bad to worse!

fiasco that could be dangerous under military circumstances. How could we back his improvement, without agreeing to overreaching?

Fortunately, I had been in similar situations countless times, because of work with my family therapy team. Adolescents and their parents almost always present this kind of problem: The kid appeals to be free, but looks like he will misuse the opportunity; the parents appeal for control, but look like they will suppress the kid altogether. The most reliable route out of this is to challenge the kid and the parents with the opposite point of view. That is, we say to the kid that his parents don't believe he can manage the opportunity, but perhaps he has some ideas about what would prove them wrong; to the parents we say that the kid thinks they have no faith in him at all, but perhaps they have some ideas about what would prove him wrong (Smith and Tiggeman, 1989; Tiggeman and Smith, 1989).

I have also found that chronic mental patients are forever posing this kind of dilemma about being free, while their caretakers are concerned about control. We replied to this man as follows: If this diagnosis of schizophrenia is correct, it is altogether improbable that you could manage a year of graduate school. Perhaps you will prove the doctors wrong? We don't know. We would be glad to reconsider a year from now. The young man was very relieved. He even volunteered that we could not lightly let him go into the military where he would be in charge of men with weapons.

A week later, he telephoned to pin me down about writing a letter for him after the academic year. This was an extremely helpful request. We had not been quite as forthright as he needed. I wrote him back to say that I did not believe the army would ever take him. Even if he had a great academic year, they could not risk a return of his psychosis, nor could we guarantee him altogether. The army is conservative. It would not serve him well to look for that kind of long shot. It would be better to prove them wrong about him in some other domain, like his graduate study, where his past history need not haunt him.

This is a critical point. I wanted to help this determined young man use his great stubbornness, but I did not want him using it where it had no chance whatsoever to help him or where it would be catastrophic. We will see if he can keep this distinction clear.

False Negatives

The opposite to the class of impossible noble causes is the class of patients who seem to be blank because they are hiding their light. Often, they have had bad experiences with our profession. Counseling in high school may have been a humiliation. Medical doctors may have blamed them for being psychosomatic. Relatives may have suggested that they were lazy for not going back to school. When your head is down from such hectoring, you may show very little of your virtue.

A Case of a Dog in Hell: Revisited after Ten Years

I described this nearly ten-year-old case in my first book (Gustafson, 1986). To make a long story short, the patient had been run down by his family as being a kind of lazy dog. I simply found that his family was wrong about him. He was extremely hardworking even when he was very depressed. In other words, he had the great American virtue of grit. He proved it by getting through a terrible grind as an undergraduate in physics, even though he liked it little.

This recognition of quality is extremely important. We have a wonderful acting company in Madison, Wisconsin, for children who perform Shakespeare (Young Shakespeare Players, directed by Richard and Anne DiPrima). The soul of the company is its pair of directors, who believe children are far underestimated and can perform great feats, and so they do. Of course, some drop by the wayside, but many respond to the challenge of remembering hundreds of lines, with their nuances and interactions. After their last performance, they ask the children to perform their favorite lines for each other by quoting Hamlet to the Players: "Come, give us a taste of your quality. Come, a passionate speech." The children respond with huge energy.

There is a limit to this recognition of quality, as my patient showed me ten years after his initial consultation, when he came for consultation twice, a year apart. He was living with his parents. He could not bring himself to stay in the temporary job market. He could not put himself on the climb up the great mountain of graduate school, because he really could not love physics. His virtue was in his art and his reading, but no one was going to pay him for his capacity to enjoy himself. He was a kind of Roman Stoic or Epicurean, living in the interstices of the Empire. Actually, was he better off in his room than he was on the Roman roads. He was very relieved that I did not press him like his parents did. I could see his quality, but I could also see it was not of this world.

THE MEDICAL SLOPE

The third slope of peril at the outset is medical, and its terrain can be summarized briefly because it has been well covered by Koranyi (1979). His opening argument could not be bettered:

> Indistinct headache or fever in a patient are never regarded by physicians as diagnostic endpoints but are viewed as a compelling demand for vigorous clinical exploration. In a similar fashion, altered mood, behavior, or perception in an individual represent equally nonspecific symptoms that require differential diagnostic scrutiny. . . . Nonspecific behavioral and mood alteration often represent the very first and, occasionally for prolonged periods of time, the one single and exclusive sign of an undetected physical illness. Flagrantly and convincingly "psychological" in nature on presentation, such masked physical conditions frequently mislead the examiner and obliterate any further medical consideration, resulting in misdiagnosis and thus, inevitably, in a treatment gone astray. (p. 414)

His study then proceeds to the evidence in 2,090 psychiatric clinic patients. Forty-three percent had one or more physical illnesses, while 46 percent of those illnesses were undiagnosed by the referring source! Self-referred and social agency–referred patients almost always had undiagnosed physical illnesses! The chief culprit was diabetes mellitus, but also common were other endocrine, nutritional, and metabolic illnesses and central nervous system and circulatory illnesses. He concludes that laboratory screening and a complete physical examination are mandatory procedures for new psychiatric patients. (See also Bartsch *et al.* [1990]; Hall *et al.* [1978, 1982]; Koran *et al.* [1989]; Muecke & Krueger [1981]; Sox *et al.* [1989]; Wells *et al.* [1989]. I am grateful to Peter Miller for these references, which essentially confirm Koranyi's findings.)

I agree completely. My one-page form (Figure 2.2) for summarizing first visits states at the very top that one-quarter of patients are likely to have undiagnosed

MEDICAL RECORD NUMBER:

NAME:

DATE OF BIRTH:

DATE:

PSYCHIATRIC EVALUATION

A. MEDICAL DIFFERENTIAL DIAGNOSIS AND RECOMMENDATIONS (All patients who have not had a medical evaluation since they have become symptomatic need to do so, as about one quarter of all psychiatric outpatients have undiagnosed and significant medical illnesses).

☐ Referall necessary ☐ Not necessary

B. PSYCHIATRIC DIFFERENTIAL DIAGNOSIS, AND RECOMMENDATIONS (All patients should understand that there is a pharmacologic therapy for nearly all psychiatric conditions, which would be the primary recommendation of most psychiatrists. Referral for this perspective is available for all patients.)

C. PSYCHOTHERAPEUTIC DILEMMA (Stated in my letter to the patient).

James P. Gustafson, M.D.
Professor of Psychiatry
University of Wisconsin Medical School

Figure 2.2. Psychiatric evaluation form.

physical illnesses and must have a medical evaluation when they become symptomatic. In fact, I am more cautious than my experience in Madison seems to warrant. My patients tend to be younger, healthier, and better off than Koranyi's in Ottawa.

Yet I have had several unforgettable experiences that I do not want to have again. The first was a foreign student anxious to get back to his home country, who, due to taking antidepressants, turned out to have no measurable blood pressure. So his anxiety had a plausible psychological cause, which might have masked an extremely dangerous physical condition. The second was a student depressed by graduate school for very adequate psychological causes, who turned out to be hypothyroid. The third was a mother who could not recover from a schizophrenic break and lapsed into the "in-the-corner lifestyle." After I interviewed her about finding some "unique outcomes" to help her, I discovered to may chagrin that she had had a concussion and a subsequent lack of concentration due to an organic brain syndrome.

Having allowed about half of the first hour for following the patient's story (Chapter 1), and about half of the first hour for sorting out the relevant dangers (Chapter 2), I am prepared to summarize my recommendations to the patient, which I will put in writing in a brief letter to the patient that follows this first interview.

In very broad strokes, I may offer no treatment, I may offer referral, or I may offer psychotherapy. I offer no treatment when the fault is malignant and the patient is not going to take responsibility. Our department remains available if there is an emergency (Malan, 1979; Weiden & Havens, 1994). If the patient wants antianxiety, antidepressant, antimanic, or antipsychotic agents, I refer him to one of my psychopharmacological colleagues. I am catholic about psychopharmacology. Some patients are comforted and improved by it, and some prefer to do without it. This is fine with me, either way. I have yet to discover that it interferes with psychotherapy, and I find it sometimes helps a patient to endure what is otherwise unendurable anxiety, depression, sleeplessness, mania, or psychosis. I suppose there are cases where it interferes, but I have not yet seen them. If the patient has a dilemma that he is prepared to work on, and I have available time, I offer psychotherapy.

Patients who do not have a basic fault (Balint, 1968) I usually offer one hour every other week. Usually, their HMO or insurance covers about twelve sessions per year, so brief psychotherapy lasts half a year. Patients who do have a benign basic fault I usually offer one hour a month. The length of psychotherapy can be indefinitely long, or can cope with the current episode only, with the opportunity to return as needed. If the patient has funding and the desire for a long journey that is slow in its curve through the unconscious, often in mid-life when the old self will no longer work and a shadow self needs to be assimilated, I usually offer one hour once a week. This is apt to continue for two to five years.

[illegible] psychotherapy.

Patients who do not have a basic fault (Balint, 1968) I usually offer one hour every few weeks. Usually, the HMO or insurance covers about twelve sessions per year, so brief psychotherapy lasts half a year. Patients who do have a benign basic fault I usually offer one hour a month. The length of psychotherapy can be indefinitely long [illegible] cope with the current episode only, with the opportunity to return as needed. If the patient has [illegible] and the desire for a long journey that it [illegible] move through the unconscious, often in mid-life when the old self will no longer work and a shallow self needs to be [illegible], I usually offer one hour once a week. This is apt to continue for two to five years.

Chapter 3

Female Dilemmas

WORKING THROUGH

The schemes of psychotherapy will be most weak in the middle, where a certain formlessness is probable in the patient, setting in motion a certain line of attack by the doctor. Freud's (1913/1963) opinion is usually accepted:

> He who hopes to learn the fine art of the game of chess from books will soon discover that only the opening and closing moves of the game admit of exhaustive systematic description. (p. 135)

Freud (1914/1963) then provides a plan of battle for the middle phase, which he calls "working through":

> The condition of the present illness is shifted bit by bit within the range and field of operation . . . which consists chiefly in translating it back again into terms of the past. (p. 162)
>
> The past is the patient's armory out of which he fetches his weapons for defending himself against the progress of the analysis, weapons which we must wrest from him one by one. (p. 161)
>
> One must allow the patient time to get to know this resistance of which he is ignorant, to "work through" it, to overcome it, by continuing the analytic rule in defiance of it. (p. 165)

Freud's metaphor is entirely military. The doctor is simply to hold fast to the analytic rule, which will wrest the weapons of the patient from him one by one, and which will accomplish the translation into terms of the past. The virtue of the recommendations is that they can be remembered when things bog down in the middle, as they usually do.

Little changes in the accounts of the next eighty years, from Reich to Alexander and French to Mann, Malan, Davanloo, and even when the analytic rule becomes the cognitive rule of exposing self-defeating thoughts or the behavioral rule of exposure to anxiety-inducing situations. The middle calls for more of the same, steadfastly.

The weakness of this universal military strategy for the middle of psychotherapy will be evident, I hope, in the following pair of consultations I did for a student of mine concerning her patient, who was stuck in the usual middle bog.

The Case of the Mythical Dimensions of J. Crew, or Letting the Bears In

The patient is an attractive female graduate student, who complains of being too dependent on her boyfriend and too little focused on herself. She clings to him, anxious and jealous of all possible rivals. This is debilitating because she has to follow him around (more mentally) to forestall his pursuit of another female and because she, therefore, cannot attend to her own business.

In this first consultation, I was impressed by the clarity of the patient and the resident. They were following the analytic rule of uncovering the dynamics of the patient's debility. They knew them very well. This did little to alter her clinging. So what was the gap in the dynamic story that drove its perpetual round?

I felt that their analytic discourse about conscious weakness was obscuring a covert strength. I proposed to the patient that we just sit a bit, and see what came up in the lull. Indeed, this was hard for her. She became restless, mocking. I noted to her that she was very uncomfortable with her superiority. She became more so, laughing at the pictures in my notes.

I then felt that the time was right for a dive into her dreams. I said to her that I bet she dreamt about all this. Indeed, she did, and the most startling dream was of a visit with her family to the funeral home where a young male friend who had died in an auto accident was being shown. As she is helped to go take a look in the casket, she reaches the culmination of the dream, which narrows down to the death mask of her friend. The mask is smiling, yet it has a crack like lightning right down the middle. Straw swirls over it, obscuring the clarity, and the dream closes.

As we went together back into the dream, she was at first comforted by the smile, but as soon as I posed the crack, she began to cry, saying she felt his sweet presence so vividly that he seemed to come toward her. She then resumed her usual composure, saying she felt embarrassed by all this feeling, which she had not experienced before about this tragic loss. I replied that she was putting the lid back on, as happens when she fears what watchers will make of her. I suggested that this was the source of her weakness, that she projected her powers onto others, especially men, and especially critical men. She obviously feared to own her own strength of feeling. Both she and the resident were impressed by her intensity. Obviously, she could bear her own strength of feeling, given company.

The resident and the patient went back to working on this, and I did not see them again for several months, until they came back for a second consultation. They explained to me that their work was going well, insofar as the patient was able to follow the resident's suggestion that she forego following her boyfriend around and pass through the anxiety of forgetting him and owning her own feelings.

Now, I had not presented such a suggestion myself. While I had proposed, indeed, that the patient's weakness came from a failure to own herself, I did not have in mind to give such a directive. The resident made that translation. While the previous marching orders had been the analytic rule of uncovering against resistance, the new marching orders had become the behavioral rule of exposure to the anxiety. This had worked somewhat, since the patient did feel less anxious about being self-possessed, instead of other-possessed. They were still in a bog.

The patient wanted to look attractive like the young goddesses in the catalog of J. Crew. Ashamed as she was of this longing, it still possessed her in many ways. She did not feel worthy, because she was not up to the ideal look, and she feared her boyfriend would eventually turn up a goddess of complete being who did feel worthy. The opening speech of Shakespeare's *Twelfth Night* is a most beautiful argument against trusting the fate of the goddess of J. Crew:

> O spirit of love, how quick and fresh art thou,
> That, notwithstanding thy capacity,
> Receiveth as the sea. Nought enters here,
> Of what validity and pitch soe'er,
> But falls into abatement and low price
> Even in a minute.
>
> * * *
>
> Yet who would miss it either? Thus,
> if music be the food of love play on.

Herein lies the dilemma of the play, and of our patient: If she had not love, she is low; if she has love and is high, she dreads to lose it. Thus, the resident's suggestion to turn away from this did not actually get it to relinquish its grip on her.

Her agitation in talking about this dilemma was striking. I noted the anxiety to her, comparing it to the drive of athletes to win contests. She replied that she is extremely competitive, yet she also wants to be in peace. I posed her dilemma. If she gave up being a goddess, she felt in danger of losing. If she did not give it up, she was in danger of losing all tranquility.

Having reached the center of her disturbance, I asked for her dreams, as I had in the first consultation. She told me that the most striking dream repeated itself, a sure sign of something big being ignored. In these dreams, she was petrified that a bear would get her. She had had these dreams even as a child. Her parents had tried to ease her fears by laughing at them. She herself now tried to laugh.

I told her she still had much to fear of bears, because she had not been allowed to own fear. It was to be covered up by an attitude of superiority (mocking and humor also strengthened her) as a kind of persona, or mask. She was really still a child in this respect. She replied so freshly, ". . . shall we let in some bears? . . . my ultimate fear." I replied that we might indeed. We went together into the dream.

The bears, she told me, were not regular bears, but ". . . mean bears, . . .

kinda checking me out." How mean? "They would rip my shirt off!" Checking you out? "Those bears are men!" This intrigued her, and made her shiver.

We were running out of her hour with me. I summarized her dilemma in my usual letter following such a consultation:

> I can be briefer and more to the point this time. You have learned a lot with your doctor about your being driven by fear of not measuring up as a goddess of J. Crew, and move increasingly toward centering on yourself and what you feel and want for yourself, especially the tranquility that is free of the frenzy of having to have others approve of you.
>
> A big part of accepting yourself is to accept your own fear as valid and as a guide to danger. This was not allowed in your family, which waved off fear, so it was a kind of cover-up of something you needed help with at five. This is why, I think, the dreams have an ancient, childlike quality, of these bears, which keep coming back.
>
> As you said so eloquently, it is time to let the bears in, to see what sets them going every several nights. Your unconscious would not send them back so often if they were not terribly important. I think you got civilized too soon, so they bring up the primitive and baleful power, like one that checks you out, to kill you.
>
> If you do not do this, I would hope you stay close to home, and look to others to judge things for you, because you would lack your own gut instinct for danger and get hurt bad (perhaps this brings us back to your friend who was killed). If you do do it, then you will have to endure becoming something of a bear yourself, who turns out to be your totem animal from the shadow side.
>
> I enjoyed talking with you very much as before, and would be glad to arrange for you to see the tapes, as you like.

FROM SINGLE TO DOUBLE PURPOSES

Dilemma as the Key Structure

The resident, like Freud, wants to march ahead to complete the journey, only she cannot get there by a straight line. She can get part way, inasmuch as her patient could go into herself and forget her boyfriend to some degree. The resident suggested she do so and bear the anxiety, and the patient was strengthened.

She cannot give up being possessed by the goddess of J. Crew, silly as it seems to her, nor can she go far into herself without running into her recurrent terror of the bear and his possession. Thus, without a better map, she is stuck indefinitely because there is great danger left and right.

In other words, she has a dilemma. A lemma is a preliminary premise, which in mathematics is used to prove theorems. A "di-lemma" occurs when there are two preliminary premises that are contradictory. One lemma is that the patient can prosper as a goddess of J. Crew. This turns out to be a life-lie (Gustafson, 1992; Ibsen, 1884) that makes her anxious, because she is not really loved for herself and can be replaced by a better model whenever such appears.

The second lemma is that she can be fully herself and loved for her full self. This turns out to be another life-lie, because she could not have her fearfulness accepted as a child, and had to pretend to be a superior adult. On the shadow slope, she is about to fall into possession of the mean bear-man, or boar. (See Hughes, 1992, for the origin of the boar as the quintessential animal of attack.)

This is a typical dilemma for an attractive woman, as Shakespeare demonstrated nearly four hundred years ago (Hughes, 1992). She is invited to contemplate herself as a goddess of complete being, like Ophelia, Desdemona, or Cordelia. This is very shaky ground to stand on, for one little fall or error in the eyes of the prince or king and she becomes the object of a death charge by the boar. All three heroines of Shakespeare die of the hero's madness.

Death may seem extreme, but actually it is not unusual. Usually, the death of the female is more gradual, as she is attended by physicians who keep her going. For instance, the very first case in a recent review of a single-session psychotherapy (Pastor, 1993) concerns a wife of a vice president married to his work, who becomes panicky when he is away and when she has to go past an intersection near her house to get to the city. She dreads the next promotion of her husband, which will send them elsewhere, and clings to her son and then to medical complaints and doctors. This lady is at the mercy of her hero's madness as well.

This is a classic dilemma for the female. Being at the mercy of the prince is terrible, but departing from him is also terrible. She is on the horns of the dilemma, as we are wont to say in everyday speech. Putting a rival on the horns of his dilemma is a medieval construction originating with Cicero (106–43 B.C.) and St. Jerome (A.D. 400) and becoming common parlance thereafter. (See Gustafson, 1995, Chapter 18.) The medieval schoolmen who loved to do it were called Cornificii by Abelard (Adams, 1907/1961, p. 303). One horn is this passive posture of the goddess of J. Crew as an admired object. The second horn is the active posture of getting angry. Both are dangerous.

It is best for the doctor to realize the double danger, or he will miss the crucial gaps in the story of the patient. In The Case of the Mythical Dimensions of J. Crew, the resident understood the drift of the patient as object, but the force of the patient as subject was unexplored, until I brought it to light as the fear of possession by bears. Although it introduces itself as a dread of being attacked that cannot be owned, I soon realized it would turn into her own attacking power in the active sense of the boar. Indeed, as soon as I suspended discussion of her debility in the form of possession by J. Crew, I got her mocking superiority.

Mastery of her dilemma means being free of possession by either extreme. She is no longer a prisoner of the belief that she has to be a J. Crew goddess to have a man. She is no longer a prisoner of boarlike rage, in the prince or in herself. Both states are

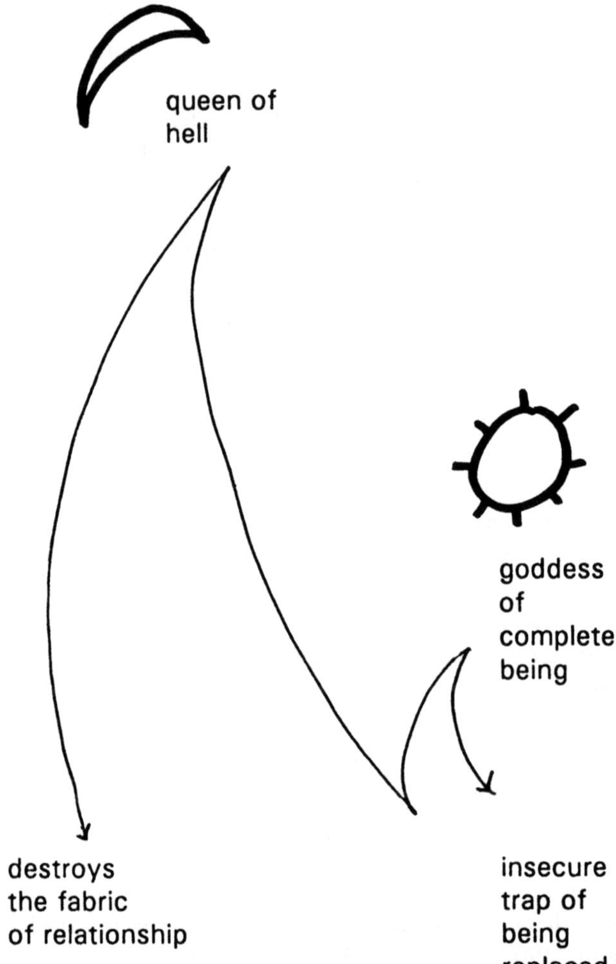

Figure 3.1. The classical white middle-class dilemma of the female as heroine.

modulated, which frees her from their ruinous consequences. She can enjoy being admired as a goddess without having to be a goddess of complete being, and she can enjoy forcefulness, without having to be a queen of hell.

I would like to add one final comment on The Case of the Mythical Dimensions of J. Crew. The dream in the patient's first consultation was of the death mask of her dead friend. Notice that the mask was smiling, with a crack running right down the middle like lightning. Now we can see it is also her own death mask, in that the smiling persona of the goddess of complete being has to be riven to let the lighting of her full presence through. As her friend seems to come sweetly toward her when we penetrate the mask in the analysis of the dream, so we also come into her full own being, with its hazards. If I were a romantic, I would welcome this full being, but I am not, and I know that she needs the vitality that comes from entering the mythical plane in shadow, yet she needs to return to the plane of reality, where J. Crew still rules the imagery of mating in her social class.

The Length of the Middle

The number of hours of psychotherapy and the number of months of experiment by the patient necessary to master the dilemma depend on its severity, the resourcefulness of the patient, and the ecology of the patient's world. The skill of the doctor also matters, for he can only guide a passage that he can undergo himself.

Classical psychoanalytic theory (Balint, 1952) recognizes two sticking positions, owing to the severity of disturbance. The first, or paranoid, position was a horn that a patient could get stuck on because of fear of letting help come close. The patient had to stay upright, vigilant, and distant, because to do otherwise with the doctor was to fall into the dark abyss of the childhood of the basic fault (Balint, 1968) with unreliable companionship that might even prove malevolent.

When the patient is in this paranoid position, there is no speeding up the help. The doctor just has to take the time to earn the trust of the patient, and dispel the negative transferences that throw such terrible images over the doctor's appearance to the patient. This may make the middle of psychotherapy long, in terms of extending it from the usual range of brief therapy in months, to long-term therapy in years. It is not necessary in all cases that long-term therapy be considered long-term when intermittent hours over a long period can allow trust to be won and thus psychotherapy to do its work. After Selvini-Palazzoli (1980), I call this long brief therapy (Gustafson, 1986).

At least half of our patients have passed the paranoid position because they have had reliable help as children, so they can let us close if we prove to know what we are doing. Thus, the patient in The Case of the Mythical Dimensions of J. Crew readily allowed me to get passed her surface persona as the smiling goddess, to her grief behind the cracked mask, and later to her fearfulness and her forcefulness as the bear or boar.

Her sticking point is the classical horn called the depressive position, upon which the patient was stuck for fear that her force would be destructive to the good she has to depend on. This is precisely her dread. She cannot enter into the force of the queen of hell, which is the boar, because it is not under her control and it will harm her chances to maintain what good she has around. The sticking point is passed only when she can allow company to enter into this forcefulness without acting it out unmercifully. I posed precisely this problem to her and her doctor in my second consultation, and she put it better than I did, as the need to let the bears in.

This for me is the great subject of brief psychotherapy: to let in the shadow side and to pass through it with company so it is modulated and mastered. Malan's (1976a,b) follow-up studies of chronic neurotics in brief psychotherapy at the Tavistock Clinic in London demonstrate that it is often possible to do this within twenty or thirty hours or even less. My own studies on a smaller scale have confirmed this (Gustafson, 1986).

DILEMMAS DO NOT GO AWAY

Motivation

This beautiful result in brief psychotherapy would be a fairy tale if its weaknesses were not admitted to. The first discussed candidly by Malan himself is in terms of motivation. The focus has to be right, but a patient must have what Malan calls motivation, the grit to bear difficult feeling, given company. Many will not, and just run away when the going gets hard. This is why I propose looking for and testing this essential capacity in the opening sessions, for we cannot do without it in the trial of the middle passage. Moran (Mike Moran, personal communication) notes that young therapists in his mental health center often take on too much of the determination that their patients lack, and end up mad at their patients for being too passive. Female patients may capitulate to their men, and thus disappoint their therapists.

Ecology

The second limitation is set by the ecology of the patient. For example, young women, like the patient in The Case of the Mythical Dimensions of J. Crew, can more readily give up neurotic clinging, and find an alternative match that respects their strength of being, when they are still in the vast shoals of schooling, where many mates are still available (for a classical example, see my Case of the Young Woman with No Self-Confidence [1986]). Middle-aged women have a much rougher time, because the mates they need as doubles for themselves are already taken. This is why they tend to stay in psychotherapy a long time with a doctor who can be the necessary company.

Ecology also governs whether there is a stage, or plane of reality, for working out a career. Some patients discover themselves on the mythical plane of their vital force, and can successfully use it to further their careers. This was the most common success in Malan's (1976a,b) study of long-term outcomes of brief psychotherapy. There is much dimming of this brilliance, however, when the patient has no love that will play in a theater that is paying handsomely. In The Case of the Dog in Hell of Chapter 2, the patient was a brilliant success in school in showing his hidden virtue, but had little success during the next ten years in the working world. This failure is commonplace and becomes more so as the economy destroys more and more sectors where good performance used to lead to a good job. The luck of the draw—being from the right family in the right and successful part of the world—has become crucial. Bourdieu (1977, 1984) calls it symbolic capital, and shows that the children of bankers in France have the best chance to become bankers, while the children of academics have the best chance to become academics.

Resolution of an Episode, and Later Episodes

The final limitation of brief psychotherapy is that the episode resolved is no guarantee of finding a way through subsequent episodes. It helps. As Malan (1976a,b) found, patients often could make their own reckoning of later episodes without the doctor if they brought to mind what he would be likely to say in the new circumstances. Thus, our patient in The Case of The Mythical Dimensions of J. Crew might free herself of clinging to her boyfriend and end her brief psychotherapy. Will she cling to the next man? If she makes a strong match, will she slip back to clinging when she has children and feels less attractive. Will she go on to find a stage in the working world where she can play at her strength, or will she merely comply in some bureaucracy? All of her later challenges have the same structural dilemma as the first, which will not go away (see Chapter 15, "Ten Follow-up Studies and the Science of Psychotherapy," for data on motivation, ecology, and the ongoing structure of dilemma).

Peter Miller (personal communication) notes that women patients in his mental health center often "can get very good access to their forceful side, sometimes at the risk of their children. It is the middle path or modulation which is hard to find and sometimes hard even for the therapist to point toward." Indeed, I find that my long-term cases are precisely those patients who take a very long time to discover, invent, and solidify a middle path. They frequently slip back into being doormats, or queens of hell. Often, they are basically faulted in the benign sense; they lack a model of balance, and are pulled under or over by huge pressures in the economic realm and by difficult men. So, there are many forces working against balance.

It turns out to be the dilemma of many females who are ambitious (Gilligan, 1982, 1990). At ten, having had good backing, they are little naturalists, fascinated by everything. By fifteen, they are out of touch with themselves, except insofar as they have a role in the adolescent pack, as did the goddess of J. Crew. By following them along year by year, between the ages of ten and fifteen, Gilligan dramatically shows that each year brings more and more responses of "I don't know" when asked how they feel about things. They increasingly become prisoners of the discourse of the local rock and roll station (Z-104). They know what Z-104 thinks, and the naturalist is lost in shadow. Whether she can be kept going, and make a big comeback in college, depends on her opportunities from parents, teachers, jobs, peers, and, these failing to some extent, psychotherapy.

Obviously, there is no single female dilemma. For example, many young women have the classical male dilemma (discussed in Chapter 4), while also having the classical white, middle-class female dilemma discussed here. Furthermore, black women have been shown to have dilemmas different from white women under certain circumstances (Ba, 1980). Social class drastically alters opportunity (El Saadawi, 1975; Bernstein, 1973). The subject of female development and its diverse pathways is a book unto itself, and even an entire field. I have compressed it here to what is most common in my practice in Wisconsin.

Chapter 4

Male Dilemmas

This chapter concerns the classic male dilemmas and the ability to fail well, which I discuss in the same breath. Why?

I have three reasons, which are the substance of this chapter. My first reason is that males in Western society run in hunting packs, which always overextend themselves and, thus, have to fail sooner or later. My second reason is that they then turn, like Shakespeare's Coriolanus, to a "world elsewhere," which, like all romances, has to fail. My third reason is that those who get past the first two failures, that is, who do not die in Rome like Coriolanus of martial madness, and who do not die in Egypt like Shakespeare's Antony of romantic foolishness, evolve only if they retain the humility to be wrong. If they lack humility, they come to a stop, and return to being pinned either to the horn of the pack or to the horn of romance.

Increasingly, females run a similar course in their careers and, therefore, this dilemma applies to them as well. Jung called it possession by the animus, Freud the dominance of the Oedipus complex. For Shakespeare it was the tragic equation (Hughes, 1992).

In proposing such scope to this chapter, I do not want to slight the technical problems of the middle of psychotherapy with males. I come precisely as I can to their dilemmas, to what they overlook, and to what we supply to help them free themselves from being dragged downhill by the neck by these archetypes.

INCREASE PACKS ALWAYS OVEREXTEND THEIR MEMBERS

The dominant male fate in Western civilization is overextending, because it is the pattern of his groups since about 1250 B.C.:

> Toward the close of the Age of Bronze and, more strongly, with the dawn of the Age of Iron (c. 1250 in the Levant), the old cosmology and mythologies of the goddess mother were radically transformed, reinterpreted, and in large measure even suppressed, by *those suddenly intrusive patriarchal warrior tribesmen* whose

> traditions have come down to us chiefly in the Old and New Testaments and in the myths of Greece. Two extensive geographical matrices were the source lands of *these insurgent warrior waves:* for the Semites, the Syro-Arabian deserts, where, as ranging nomads, they herded sheep and goats and later mastered the camel; and, for the Hellenic-Aryan stems, the broad plains of Europe and south Russia, where they had grazed their herds of cattle and early mastered the horse. (Campbell, 1964, p. 7; my italics)

Since these fellows gained momentum, they have been very difficult to stop. Greed gets a license and is only driven harder by dread of the other guys taking its supplies.

This is the engine or dynamic that heats up nearly every group of men (Levi-Strauss in Charbonnier, 1969). Those who will succeed must show that they can drive themselves harder and farther and longer, while those who do not are put to shame. This is true in Forbes Magazine, in medical school, and in politics.

Canetti's (1962/1981) term for the "suddenly intrusive patriarchal warrior tribesmen" of Campbell and the "hot engines" of Levi-Strauss is for me the most precise, and this is what he calls "the increase pack," which "is of immense importance, being the specific propelling force behind the spread of men" (p. 107). My argument is that the specific propelling force behind the spread of men is what overextends and routinely goes too far.

A Routine Case of Raging Bull

A middle-aged attorney was the last son of a hard-driving immigrant father who belittled him. He tried very hard to please the old man, but he never could. In turn he took out his exasperation on whatever he could lay his hands on, and thus became a raging bull himself, a member in full standing of that enormous totem clan.

Driven by such furious juice, he did well and got a practice that never stopped growing. Naturally, everyone wanted this bull to charge their legal enemies, and so he did, only he could not stop at the end of the day. When he got home and his wife handed over the keys to the household and the three children and the cupboard for him to make supper, there was great trouble afoot.

Here we arrive at a dangerous slope, where the bull cannot help charging downhill at his own wife and children. His very virtue in the legal world knows no boundaries, as the advertisements say for Merrill-Lynch of Wall Street, and he overruns his own family and destroys the very ground that has kept him going.

Often these patients come when it is too late, as in tragedy, because they have already done too much harm and, therefore, will never be taken back. He had just begun to frighten the children when his wife came in to tell me she was at the very edge of the precipice. Here was his last chance not to drive her over it with her children.

I knew that his only chance lay in his admitting that he had no control when he arrived home with the hairs standing up on the back of his neck. By then it was too late to manage himself. No ingenious doctor was soon going to alter his temper, which would run away with him down that incline. Therefore, I told him and his wife that "contingency plans" (White, 1989) had to intercept the bull before he got to that slope and plunged down it out of control. First, the law firm had to loosen its grip on him by about half. Second, because the first measure would fail on some days, he needed to go somewhere else after work before going home. Third, because the second measure would fail on some days, he needed an exit plan if he found himself boiling in his own kitchen. Only if he set up these precautions in advance could we even have the chance to work together in my office to extricate him from his possession by this god the bull.

Overextending in Endless Variations or Clans

Now, the bulls are but one clan of countless numbers. Really, it is no accident that the great basketball team from Chicago is one expression of the bullishness of America. It is an excellent charge, until it gets you into the stockyards.

There are badgers, wolverines, hawkeyes, and gophers, and so forth. I will use many cases in this chapter to illustrate these totemic variations that run away with my patients by their very success.

Freud certainly knew about these forces, and he described them in his case of Little Hans, the Rat Man, and the Wolf Man—males captured by becoming transformed into one of these animals. Freud ended up saying that all males are possessed, more abstractly, by the Oedipus complex. By 1923, in *The Ego and the Id* he codifies this Oedipus formulation that he had been employing more loosely for twenty years. Thus, the horse, rat, and wolf are all stand-ins for the father. By this line of thought, we could also reduce the whale in Melville's *Moby-Dick.* Ahab is only beset with revenge at his father, who would not let him have his mother at sea.

I find Canetti's argument more compelling. It has several steps. The first is that man is terribly vulnerable in small numbers, so he needs to increase himself to get game and to defend himself from hostile hordes: "Man's weakness lay in the smallness of his numbers" (Canetti, 1981, p. 108). This is true now as it was then, for the men without allies are cut out by the mergers that take over the markets. The second step is the transformation, by which men make themselves, symbolically, into the plentiful creatures that they depend upon for their supply. Thus, the Mandan tribe relied on buffaloes:

> Buffaloes, it is known, are a sort of roaming creature, congregating in huge masses, and strolling away about the country from east to west, or from north to south, or just where their whims or strange fancies may lead them; and the Mandans are sometimes, by this means, most unceremoniously left without anything to eat. . . . In any emergency of this kind, every man musters and brings out of his lodge his mask (the skin of a buffalo's head with the horns

> on), . . . and then commences the buffalo dance for the purpose of making "buffalo come." . . . The Mandan know from experience that a crowd grows and attracts into its orbit everything of the same kind which is near; whenever there is a large number of buffaloes together, more buffaloes approach. (Canetti, 1981, pp. 111–112)

The third step of Canetti's argument is that this dynamism of transformation becomes so compelling that it is capable of complete abstraction, such as we find in students who are desperate to increase grade points, salesmen their sales, academics their papers, garbage collectors their garbage, astronomers their galaxies. St. Exupery (1943) parodies this as the chief activity of "les grandes personnes," that is, adults. It is ancient, says Canetti, as in Australian aborigines:

> But what are we to say when we encounter people who designate scorpions, lice, flies or mosquitoes as their totem . . . for such creatures are plagues for the aborigine as they are for us. . . . The man who is descended from a mosquito-totem wants his people to become as numerous as mosquitoes (Canetti, 1981, p. 110)

In summary, Canetti (1981) states: "It was through the development of transformation that he really became man; it was his specific gift and pleasure" (p. 108). Thus, the first horn of a male dilemma is his specific gift and pleasure for transforming himself into the object of his pursuit, like grades, money, fame, whatever. He becomes so identified that he becomes grades, money, reputation, etc. He talks its very language, or its language talks through him.

The Case of the Rat Man

Freud (1909) wrote of this patient: "In his obsessional deliria, he had coined himself a regular rat language. . . . Little by little, he translated into this language the complex of money interests which centered around his legacy to himself" (p. 213). *Raten* is linked to *Ratten* in German, as rats are to installments. *Speilratte* are gambling debts, *heiraten* is to marry, and so forth.

I think Freud provides us here with the evidence for Canetti's argument. While it is true that the patient is obsessed with taking over from his father, his father's place is literally in the rat-totem of corrupt German commerce. The patient's survival is to transform himself into a rat, so he can increase his installments or *Ratten,* and get pals for gambling or *Spielratte,* and marry a rat-wife or *Heiraten,* thereby generating a long line of rats or *Raten.* In brief, he belongs, and thus he prospers, in the increase pack of the rat. Of course, the first horn of his dilemma as an emerging rat is that he overextends his rat activities so he is in a frenzy to have everything, and cannot bear the frustration set up by so much greed. Thus, he is a typical male.

He is unusual in his genius for language; most of my males so captured are less inventive in their talk, but merely mouth the platitudes of the pack they belong to—of sport, of medicine, of whatever.

The Case of the Stern Eye of Max Weber

A successful yet entirely typical young businessman grew up in the cloud of his grandfather's fundamentalist presence, graduated to the secular accomplishments that grew naturally out of the Protestant work ethic and evolved into the spirit of capitalism (Weber, 1958) in his parents, and was lost by twenty-five as if he were in an empty sea lacking moral purpose.

I told him that his god had broken down, and that we would have to wait for light from his unconscious for a way forward. His first dream was very beautiful in its economy and its whimsy: He dreamt he went to sea in a boat, from which he struck golf balls. He laughed and commented that it was surely sub-par golfing, which was a relief from being driven under the stern eye of Max Weber. I commented that first dreams often spell the fear of dreaming, so he likely feared that I too could be unmerciful. Then, he wept, and dropped his loud voice and his double-time pace, which was making him ill.

The Case of "Thomas Merton"

Some increase packs are humble, but the humility itself runs away with the man. Some are delaying, like academics in the library, so the delay itself runs away with the man. Often, these packs are in revulsion of the openly greedy.

Thomas Merton (1948) lost his father when he was sixteen and plunged into a riot of pleasures. It was not very long before this experiment lost its center and seemed a meaningless carnival at the University in Cambridge:

> Above all, why did the very boisterousness of the soccer blues, the rugger players, the cricketers, the oarsmen, the huntsmen and drinkers in the Lion and the clumsy dancers in the Rendezvous—why was all their noise so oafish and hollow and ridiculous? It seemed to me that Cambridge and, to some extent, the whole of England was pretending, with an elaborate and intent and conscious, and perhaps in some cases a courageous effort, to act as if it were alive. And it took a lot of acting. It was a vast and complicated charade . . . . (p. 141)

Like St. Augustine long before him, Merton turns to Christ for purpose and finds it in His merciful love as a check against all selfish and trivial gratification. It is an old story.

My patient had followed this ancient road and become a devoted teacher of philosophy, who gave as much to his students as anyone I ever saw. Like Merton, he believed in reason and in compassion. I saw him two years into his pursuit of a beautiful young woman, a fellow teacher, who eluded him. She was obviously wounded, because she kept apart from everything but her classroom.

He wooed her, but he just couldn't get very far. She would go out with him, but then she wouldn't answer her telephone for a week. She would make love, but she wouldn't talk about herself. She would jog with him, but she wouldn't have lunch.

For two years, she held this precise distance. I told him that it was evident to me that she needed to be half in and half out. She would not give up. Very gradually hints came of what lay behind her persona. A few words about an eating disorder, psychosis, and even rape drifted in from the past. I do not think much of this registered on him until one day he waited for her on her bed. Two hours later she came out from under it and told him she had been terrified he was out to kill her.

Even then, he wanted to save her. He so believed in Christ's compassion because it had saved him. It must know no limits. Surely, God could not let this woman perish without aid. Thus he reasoned with her, to no avail. This is what I mean by overextending in the name of love, a most common horn for the males of the species.

THE HORN IN SHADOW

Once I came to the conclusion that the second, or shadow, horn is more dangerous than the first, or obvious, horn, I was able to make much more sense out of the male dilemmas. The shadow horn was always missing from the story, yet it governed the man unaccountably. He persisted on the first, in what seemed a senseless drifting into overextension.

A Case of the Perfect Politician

This man was just what we need in the Capitol. He is a public servant, par excellence, who will pass the laws that defend our wilderness, our children, and our economy. No one keeps the light on later to finish a draft of a bill, a speech, or a memorandum dispatching his subordinates to key battles. He is exhausted. Not one increase pack, but twelve different causes run away with him as their hostage.

He could see where this was going. He could not keep it up. He could not get out of it either. He only could say no by sending the supplicant to his appointments' secretary, who might not have room for a while on the schedule. Then he might be lucky to get out of something, but never directly. He came to me, because he was alarmed to discover he was thinking about suicide as a way of getting out of this brilliant career.

Thinking as I am wont, I posed to him this liberal's dilemma. If he was going to be everyone's savior, he was going to be ruined. If he declined this slope, and did something more modest, there was a chance. I guessed there was some huge danger in that direction. I proposed that he draft a memorandum for himself about what he would pare down to, as most important. I told him I did not think he could actually do it, but I did not yet know why.

Indeed, he could not do it all at once, but he did begin to cut away at the harnesses that were dragging him down, starting by getting a new appointments' secretary who did not give him away so readily. The astounding thing was this. After one of these middle sessions, where he was freeing himself, he was struck like St.

Paul by lightning, throwing him back twenty years. He had refused his father, also a politician, a visit, and then, coming belatedly, found him dead—a suicide. We had begun to understand his terror of going his own way.

The Banality of Evil

Ordinarily, the danger on the shadow horn is less dramatic, if still very bad. The man sees his work going nowhere and dreams of a world elsewhere, which turns out to be worse than nowhere.

A Case of Small Business

I will be schematic about this story because it is just that—schemes that do not live up to their promises. As a traveling salesman, our subject got more and more tired. In retrospect, it was not so bad, because he would refresh himself by going fishing, going to ball games, and horsing around with his children. Mondays were hard to start up again.

He got the bright idea of becoming his own boss selling sporting goods. The great American god of small business had taken him over; he was full of energy once more. This clouded his judgment, as gods do when they surround you with their purposes. He mortgaged everything they had, achieved half the capital he needed, and worked until ten o'clock every night for ten years, and made a go of it, but just held even, and finally collapsed.

Western Mythology

It is startling what you can see once you get an eye for the usual gods and what they wreak. It helps to have had a liberal education in things like Christianity, medieval love, and Renaissance capitalism, for these things are still what inspire us. These masks of God (Campbell, 1964) have a secular veneer, but this is thin and religious power readily shows through.

A Case of Henry the Fifth

A man strode into my office like the military commander that he indeed was—brisk, decisive, and, perhaps, a little flagging. I could see that in his sad eyes. From a childhood where he was utterly alone on the farm he had made himself a leader of men. (This is a variation on *Citizen Kane,* or orphan turned publisher.)

His sadness was this. In his driving forward, he had worn out his wife. After thirty years, she had had too much of his forceful views about every side of their enterprise, and had gone off to a kind of nunnery to live in peace. He went to appeal to her in her tower, where he sat at her foot and courted her as of old. She would not come down to go back into the world with him, love him as she did, for she knew she would surrender her weaker will to his again. Only Shakespeare's Kate could stand up to a Henry like him, and she lacked the vitality.

This was extremely difficult for him to comprehend. After all, when you have led an English army of five hundred to defeat a French army of five thousand at Agincourt, what is the refusal of a weak woman? He did not get it. But he was losing heart after two years, which finally brought him to me.

I told him that his kingdom was empty without his queen. The plane of reality was no match for him, but it was lusterless without his goddess. Therefore, he was a troubadour. He asked me, I thought rhetorically, whether there was danger that way? Yes, I replied, it wasn't going to work, hard as that might be for his willful self to comprehend. I did not think it could be given up, altogether, because troubadours do not give up just because their cause is a losing one. No, it is their glory to continue forever, in the service of the divine lady. They live by the light of the moon, not in the dull sun.

TACKING BETWEEN THE PLANE OF REALITY AND THE MYTHICAL PLANE

If the plane of reality is going to be dull, and if the mythical plane is going to be impossible, why not tack back and forth from one plane to the other? I do think that it is the best chance for happiness we have in this world, but it is more readily said than done. To meet a test, we easily tack too far into the plane of reality, and are stuck. We readily tack too far into the mythical plane and strike the very moon, and fall headlong out of the sky. There are great pulls of gravitation, earthly and lunar, which will shipwreck us if we do not have a map and thus see them before they get a grip on us.

Peter Miller (personal communication) reminds me that this tacking is more readily said than done because the forces are often too much to bear. Many men in his mental health center have been downed and can't get up to fight again on the plane of reality: "They dwell quite firmly in a world elsewhere or in hell." This is like the classical female dilemma, which reverses the horns of the classical male dilemma: hoping to be admired, they can be hellish when they are not. Thus, they wait quite passively. Those few who can still do battle also face long odds, for "small miscalculations can ruin a person, and . . . they need somehow to find the *courage* to be *wrong again.*"

A Case of Crossing the River Jordan

A doctor worked hard in the medical establishment, wearing himself out as a junior faculty, and longed to go west to set up his own clinic in a faraway place. I will give just a few images from his epic dream about this big change.

He began, sitting astride his bicycle, in a huge and perfect garden. He took a right turn and came to a great river, which had a little bridge. To the left of the

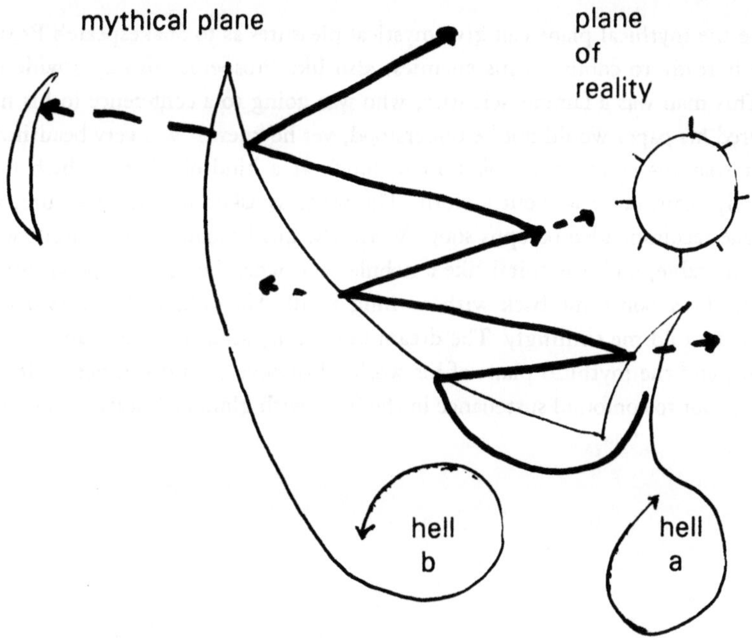

Figure 4.1. The classical dilemma of the male as hero.

bridge were two cars, an old Ford and a Mercedes-Benz, the latter face down in the mud. He went down to take a closer look and saw two snakes upon the water, yellow-brown, coiled, but in the vertical plane, springing forward with suddenness. One struck him hard in the neck, and he awoke.

To be brief, the Mercedes-Benz had been hurled into the ground by a kind of Zeus enraged, himself possessed, when he allowed himself to be subordinate to the medical chiefs in such cars. The crashing blow to his neck alluded to his mythical and boyhood days on the baseball field, when some pitcher would go for his head. He was duly warned.

If he went west and bound himself again, for his success on the plane of reality, to the worldly and local powers, he would swerve wildly away into myth. If, however, he just followed his innocent curiosity, like a Lydgate (Eliot, 1865) in love with natural observation, he would, again, be struck down as in his boyhood by men who play hard and for keeps. He was specifically warned about tacking too far onto the plane of reality, by compromise, and so he was specifically warned about tacking too far onto the mythical plane, by curiosity.

A Case of Octopus Soup

Finally, it is sometimes possible for our patients to mature to the point that they no longer have to invest earthly work or women with mythical powers. This is helpful because the mythical plane can give mystical pleasures as to Shakespeare's Prospero, yet he is ready to confound his enemies, also like Prospero, with eyes wide open.

This man was a famous scientist, who was going to a conference in his honor. He feared his paper would not be understood, yet he knew it was very beautiful. He dreamt that his colleagues took him to lunch at a kind of bistro, which had an extremely plain table without a cloth. The waitress asked him his pleasure, and a colleague recommended octopus soup. When the girl brought it, it floated two feet above the table, and was spiral like a nebula, and when he put his spoon into it to taste it, the spoon came back with nothing at all. He woke and understood it at once, as he told me smilingly. The dream beautifully separated the plane of reality, so plain, and the mythical plane of his world of discovery, so magnificent. It would be better not to confound sustenance in the first, with glorious beauty in the second.

Chapter 5

Sharp Endings

I will be brief in this chapter on sharp endings, and in the next on loose endings, because I believe there is little to say about them, and do in them, if at the outset I have properly set up for a journey that can reach its destination, and if I carry out my mapping in the middle to guide the patient through the horns of his or her dilemma. We part at the end with no great ceremony, because I am no longer needed.

Ordinarily, I agree to be summoned back when I am needed again, so there is no need for a tragic parting over a marvelous relationship that is going to be lost forever (Malan, 1979, Chapter 16; Mann, 1973). Like Freud (1937/1963), I do not believe that central conflicts or dilemmas get settled once and for all in a given period of a patient's life: "For, if the instincts are causing disturbances it is a proof that the dogs are not sleeping and if they really seem to be sleeping we have not the power to wake them" (p. 249). Continuing in Freud's metaphor, I aim to settle the dogs in a particular episode of the patient's life, assuming that they will wake again later, and I may well be needed three or four times altogether (Bennett, 1985) over thirty years. But the subject of loose endings is for the next chapter.

Here I discuss sharp endings. They do occur in tragic form, usually because of a prior assessment error. They also occur in a more ordinary form, because many patients like to break off completely from dependence and because many patients leave the vicinity to start over in a new place.

THE TRAGIC FORMS OF ENDING

I see fewer and fewer of these awful situations as I get better at reading what is needed during the first session. I have certainly learned the hard way—from starting off with patients on impossible projects. When I had to call them off, I had to bear the pain and rage I caused in the patient and my own guilt for having misled the patient about what we would accomplish. This is extremely unpleasant.

The simplest errors are with patients who delay finishing something or facing something, like school, or a weakness in work, or anxiety in social life. They talk about facing it, but they do not do it. We doctors who propose to talk further are a natural stopping place for them. We blunder, as Alexander and French (1946) put it, if we agree to their "couch diving" with us. We are thus in collusion. When we wake up to this and tell the patients, they rightly blame us for not telling them before! Of course, they do not like to be told at the outset either, but at least we have spared them wasted ventures.

A Case of a Bumbler

This man would make a mess of anything, and so he did—of marriages, children, friends, extended family, and construction work. He was very bright, but a bumbler. I got involved with him ten years ago, as a noble cause for realizing his potential. He was of a family of high standing.

I did help him for a while. He got free of a punishing wife, and he stopped letting his teenagers run all over him. He had terrible work habits, and he would take to bed and let his place go to hell. This got his prestigious family all over his case and all over me. I did not like it a bit.

The truth was that he could putter around and that was about it. He was not about to become a competent carpenter at the age of fifty. Even if he improved some, he would be hopelessly outclassed by the young, vigorous, and dedicated competition.

As this began to become obvious to me, he began to develop ailments—back pain, weight gain, headaches. Naturally he claimed disability. This put me in a very awkward position.

I could see that his body didn't work too well, but I could also see that his complaints were a dodge from having to compete when he could not compete. His medical doctor saw it the same way. Neither of us wanted to be in collusion with medical excuses.

I basically told the patient as much, and he flew into a rage. Fortunately, he fired me. Yet it was all very ugly. If I could do it all over again, I would tell him at the outset that I did not think he was going to take care of business. I would be willing to be proven wrong, yet I would leave that to him and not to me. I see many like him, and I have it out with them as soon as possible.

The delay stories seem tragic to their protagonists, and to their families, but they are actually tragicomedies, because the outcome is obvious to the trained eye at the outset.

Disasters

Some disasters move us deeply, because they involve the patient's longing to be looked after. We do it by listening, but the patient is never able to fulfill the longing in the world, and then we leave him. Then he really goes to pieces.

A Case of a "Wolf Man"

This middle-aged man was as appealing as Freud's (1918/1975) own Wolf Man and just as entitled. He got very involved with one of our residents for two years, the resident becoming the patient's savior from his family of successful and cold technocrats. I heard about the case from supervising the resident.

He came into psychotherapy after losing a beautiful girlfriend in college who loved him, the ugly prince. Her warmth saved him first, the resident second. The patient was in constant contemplation of his lost girlfriend and would talk of little else. These monologues were tedious, and the resident dreaded the visits. He hit upon the device of telling the patient that he had six months of psychotherapy to go, whereupon the resident would leave and the patient would be on his own. In this maneuver, he followed Freud's precedent with the Wolf Man. If he had studied the later history of the case, he might have thought twice. Freud's Wolf Man did bow to ending, but later took revenge by obliging Freud, who had made him a famous case, to look after him financially! Freud took up collections for him, and later arranged a second and violent analysis for him with Ruth Mack Brunswick (Garner, 1971).

In any event, the resident's patient took his dismissal with little show of feeling, continuing his monologues much the same. He then proceeded to rob several banks, and ended up in prison. The wolf came out and had his way after all.

Entitlement

I have seen this tragic sequence a few times in twenty years. There are several necessary elements. The first is a terribly injured and appealing child in the patient. The second is some miracle of rescue, often performed previously in the patient's life by a special teacher, friend, or ally, and then resumed in psychotherapy. The third is the complete absence of any chance to have this miracle occur again. The patient isn't going to win over anyone if, like Freud's Wolf Man, he is obsessed with oral, anal, and genital perversions or, like A Case of a "Wolf Man," he is a tedious cataloguer of his long-lost girlfriend's virtues.

The stalemate goes on in psychotherapy as long as the doctor can stand it, and as long as the doctor stays in town. The tragedy occurs when the break finally comes. It takes the form of an antisocial attack, like bank robbing, or a direct suicidal attack.

I once got a patient of the latter kind from a graduating resident who assured me the patient was an excellent candidate for psychotherapy. The patient was profoundly suicidal, and I ended up talking to her on the telephone for fifteen minutes nearly every night for half a year before she could spare herself.

From this experience I learned always to make my own assessments and to tell referring parties that the patient needs to have several names so that I am not in the position of being the only and last hope. Then I am freer to give back some responsibilities to the patient who works with me, so it is not my terrible burden.

ORDINARY FORMS OF ENDING

Ordinarily, sharp endings occur when the patient moves to another part of the country or the patient wants to resume independence in town. These are variations of the pioneer spirit, of moving on and of self-reliance. My job is to pose the hazards of the frontier.

A Case of Passing Over the Bar

A woman in her mid-thirties came to me when she discovered her husband cheating on her with another woman. This experience led by association to some terrible experiences she had had as a child with her father. She was also sick of working in a bureaucracy and having little adventure in life. Her life had never taken off, because she married out of high school and had always worked in the insurance business.

The most striking thing about her was how her face could gain or lose twenty years in a flash. The tedious and commonplace story of her entrapment in the ordinary made her look fifty-five, while the urge to see the world made her look fifteen. Was there some way to be thirty-five?

I had been seeing her about once a month, in the long brief therapy I often use with HMOs that grant twelve sessions a year, because I thought she needed several years to make a very big turnaround. I did not think she needed more sessions with me than one a month.

After a year and a half, she was clear about how she had been fooled by her husband. She decided she was ready to start over, and she would go West, as a teacher. Thereupon, we had seven sessions to come to a close before she departed. Essentially, it would be a new beginning (Balint, 1968).

My problem with the last seven sessions was to give her as sound a map as I could for her journey. Actually, her unconscious already had the map, so all I needed to do was to pose back to her from her dreams the problems she had to cope with to stay clear of peril.

On the very threshold of leaving her husband, she dreamt of looking back at him. In profile, he looked young. When she came closer, and looked him in the face, he was ancient. Of course, these were the two faces that she tended to wear herself. Then the dream looked forward to a beach on the Pacific Ocean where women were bathing. Two men in a boat were preparing to leave the beach for the open sea. They proceeded to plow through the women, smashing one after another, as she watched in horror from the beach.

This is a Janus dream, looking backward and forward, linking up the past and future. It warned her: "Look, you didn't look closely at your husband; in your innocence you thought him young like you, and actually he was possessed by an ancient archetype that plows through women." Interestingly, a previous dream had been about looking down from a hill at a tidepool, where men on a raft were drowning women in stagnant water, while a beautiful ocean liner loomed over the sandbar. This one warned: "Oh, you want to leave the stagnant and old waters, do you? You are going to go over the bar? You'd better be watchful for the beach!"

She can pass over the bar only if she can be both young and old simultaneously. If she is only young, she will be amazed by evil. If she is old, she will lack vitality for the sea. So the young face is one horn that will catch her, and the old face is the other horn. Can she see with two different eyes, and thus have an adequate and double description of the world?

Her final two sessions and dreams answered as follows. In the second to last she was wearing a bathrobe, and reached down to tie the sash, only to be startled by her hands being full of scissors, knives, and even hedge shears! This dream led to two big subjects: her grief about cutting many ties in leaving and her rage at men who might misuse her again.

In her final dream, she dreamt she was a deer looking west out on to a beautiful meadow, which was circled on the near side by a road with a single car coming

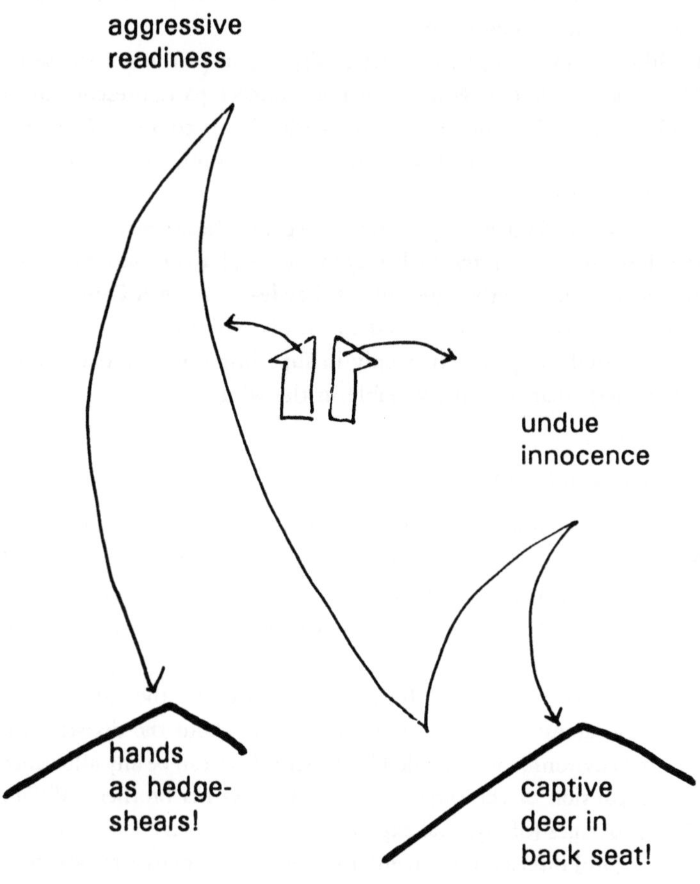

Figure 5.1. The ongoing dilemma of passing over the bar.

toward her. It was a jalopy. She got into the back seat, even as a deer, but could not get out. Struggling, she did get out, and went through the trees to an old house like the one of her childhood. She felt great fear, both for getting into the jalopy and not being able to get free, and for going back into her father's house.

Her last two dreams show her tacking between aggressive readiness for the new plane of reality and going too far, and undue innocence, going too far into the back seat with a man. These, indeed, are the two great excesses to which she is liable. These are the horns of her ongoing dilemma in going from east to west. I helped her find her way through the pass, by posing the problems left and right.

Problem-Posing

I like to end with pictures, especially dream pictures, because they stay with the patient better than words, which fade quickly. Pictures can be contemplated. I still have several from my own analysis twenty years ago that are as vivid as ever in my mind's eye so I can keep returning to them. By contrast I don't recall anything that my analyst actually said to me.

I also like to end with pictures, especially dream pictures, because I can, like Freire (1970), pose problems with them that connect past, present, and future. I want to look through these pictures at the world that is coming. Thus, the patient and I together assume that it will be difficult, feel its difficulty, and consider a path that is altogether probable between the horns.

Finally, I like to end with pictures, especially dream pictures, because I get back a very beautiful and individual imagination and a collision with the plane of reality. My patients need both, especially as they leave. As in A Case of Passing Over the Bar, they otherwise grow wearily old on the plane of reality, and remain fresh but childish on the mythical plane. It is only in superimposing the two planes that we get something new that is actually viable in the world.

A Case of an American Writer

It is often not possible for patients to superimpose the two planes. If I half open my study window, I get a beautiful glimpse of the back of the house perpendicular to the back of the house. I cannot live there. The optical illusion vanishes, as soon as I move my head too far. The backside picture has a very thin insertion into the plane of reality.

According to Poirier (1966), this is the usual case for the American writer, for example, Henry James: "In one sense his novels are about the disaster of assuming that within the environments provided by society there can be any allowance of space for the free expansion of the inner self" (p. 32). As his brother, William James, wrote: "[The] passages [of mystical experience that have] an enormous sense of inner authority . . . [are] inserted into an environment which refuses to bear them out for

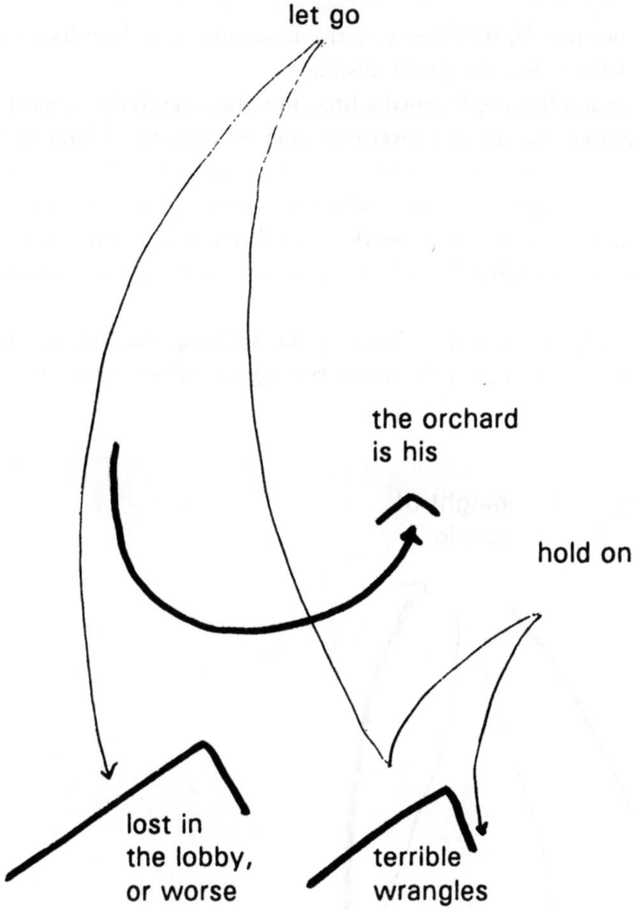

Figure 5.2. The ongoing dilemma of an American writer.

any length of time" (pp. 14–15). So "The greatest American authors really do try, against the perpetually greater power or reality, to create an environment that might allow some longer existence to the hero's momentary expansions of consciousness" (p. 15). Thus, Mark Twain's Huck Finn has a beautiful, free passage with Jim on the Mississippi.

My patient had two such passages. I saw him but six visits. He came because he was very tense about his one and only son, the son being thirty-five and very caught up on Wall Street. His wife told him he was meddling in his son's business, and ought just to let him go. Indeed, father and son had had a falling out that preoccupied this father.

He could not let go, for the passage of childhood with this boy had been the freest expression of his own life, this Jim getting much from this Huck, and vice versa. Huck was now on Wall Street, in the usual tangles, and not liking interference from Jim anymore. Jim was pretty distraught.

His grief and fretting lessened a little in telling me about it, most poignantly when I understood that he had never had much of a childhood himself. I could not hold back a tear myself when he told me how he and his father watched from the little corner left of the family farm while the foreclosers bulldozed their beautiful orchard. From then on it was all work. I could feel how precious it was to him to get a childhood, secondhand and later through his son, and how terrible it was to give it up.

He was very shy. It was evident from his shuffling feet that he would stay no longer than necessary and run the risk of wearing out his welcome. Seeing as we had

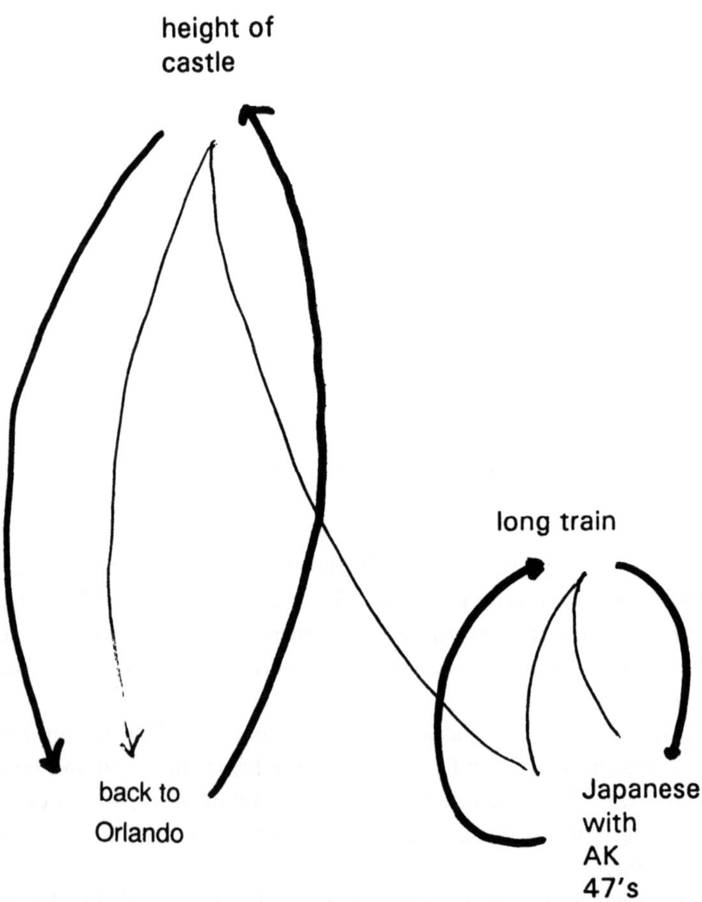

Figure 5.3. The ongoing dilemma of crossing the River Jordan.

already had three hours together, he was restless, but gave me a very clear dream of his predicament in letting go of his son.

He dreamt he was standing halfway up the sticky steps in a theater when a nondescript female with sticky lipstick came up to him and kissed him unpleasantly. He saw into her oral cavity, as though through pressed glass. His wife smiled and pretended not to notice. Finding himself next in the lobby, he could neither go back into the theater, nor out into the cold, pouring rain. This predicament brought tears to his eyes.

I told him it was very painful to give up his theater with his son, to fear falling in love in a different theater, and to be left in a public lobby. I could see, given this, why it was so hard for him to let go of his son.

The reply from his dream in the penultimate and fifth session was simply that he found himself back in the orchard. He told me everything about it, and I was extremely moved. I told him he belonged to it and it to him forever, and nobody could ever take it from him. We found a second passage with, in James's words, "an enormous sense of inner authority."

It was his alone, and would, perhaps, never again be inserted into the world. In the sixth and last session, he was still astounded by the power of the fifth, and we ended.

A Case of Crossing the River Jordan, Again

Some patients have further prospects in the world after ending with me, like the doctor I described in A Case of the River Jordan in Chapter 4. The reader may recall his fear of his own violence when trapped, and his fear of the violence of other men.

I will describe one other dream of his, one that gives me faith in his abilities to watch out for himself. He dreamt he was on a long train of a successful journey, yet it was a lie, because Japanese with AK-47 rifles were firing all along into one of the compartments. The journey over, a parade in celebration, and a climb up a tower in a beautiful castle with Persian rugs led to a great open window. Then he had to go back to Orlando, Florida.

The beauty of the dream was that it was circular. After he ascended to heaven, he came back down to the most banal of cities, starting over. And it was as if he circled over the train itself, watching the firing squad from in its midst. He refused to believe in arriving, and this is what convinced me that he would stay alert.

[illegible]

[illegible]

[illegible]

[illegible]

[illegible]

[illegible] enemy, yet it was a lie, because Japanese with AK-47 rifles were firing all along into one of the compartments. The journey over, a parade in celebration, and a climb up a tower in a beautiful castle with Persian rugs led to a great open window. Then he had to go back to Orlando, Florida.

The beauty of the dream was that it was circular. After he ascended to heaven, he came back down to the most banal of cities, starting over. And it was as if he circled over the train itself, watching the firing squad from in its midst. He refused to believe in arriving, and this is what convinced me that he would stay alert.

Chapter 6

Loose Endings

Most of my patients in brief psychotherapy end loosely with me, in the sense that they have no further need of me now, but might later. They have gotten through a difficult passage, such as getting fired or divorced, or losing confidence in themselves, with myself as company. We conclude the episode.

I am the general practitioner (Balint & Norell, 1973) who will be around when needed, or the mentor in college or graduate school who can be pulled back in. In this respect, I am taking up the role, vacated by the family doctor, and filled, increasingly, by the department of psychiatry in a health maintenance organization (Bennett, 1983, 1985).

COMPLETE PSYCHOTHERAPY

It is a nice idea that psychotherapy can be so profound that the patient meets all further emergencies in his life by himself or with his network. Long-term psychotherapies, like psychoanalysis, purport to achieve this ideal. Sometimes they do. Sometimes they don't. Shapiro (1976) found that 55 percent of the graduates of the William Alanson White Institute, all of whom had undergone psychoanalysis, sought further treatment (quoted in Bennett, 1983). I have many patients in long-term psychotherapy who are working on this kind of project of complete readiness for life's ups and downs.

Bateson (1979) calls it Learning III, in contrast to Learning Zero, I, or II. Learning Zero is when the patient repeats the error. Learning I is when he finds a new solution. Learning II is when he learns an entire category or set of related problems, and solves the entire set. Learning III is when he is engaged in the continual discovery that any set of solutions has its limitations and, therefore, must be overturned.

Learning I is common, and is the aim of solution-focused psychotherapy. This has been popularized by the Ericksonian school, among others, as a challenge to more formless or aimless methods (De Shazer, 1987). Learning II is often possible, and is the aim of dynamic psychotherapy. This has been popularized by the psychodynamic school, among others, as a challenge to treatment for only symptomatic improvement (Malan, 1976a,b, 1979). The test of dynamic change is whether an entire class of difficult circumstances, which previously made the patient symptomatic and disturbed, is now handled with adaptive new solutions and not just with withdrawal from the trouble.

Learning III is very unusual, I think, and I know of no research that had the concept or its equivalent and went looking to see whether it occurred from psychotherapy or not. It is the chief characteristic of original artists and scientists and other mortals who are forever developing an antithesis, as Hegel would have it, to their present thesis, and thus arriving at a new synthesis—which drives a new antithesis, and so on.

Obviously, some few have learned to do this, with or without psychotherapy, as the biographies and autobiographies of some of the famous will attest. It is less known how humbler persons have achieved these histories as well. There are a few examples in Studs Terkel's (1972) huge series of interviews of hundreds of working people, such as "The Mason, Carl Murray Bates" (pp. 17–22). Most of the subjects just went flat in their work to survive at all. There is no sharp distinction between Learning II and III, as many go through major transformations many times in their lives, as in college, marriage, childbirth, and so on. They just may not work on it on a daily basis like an artist (Ruth Gustafson, personal communication).

I believe that brief psychotherapy can, occasionally, supply what is necessary for the path of Learning III, and sometimes a series of brief psychotherapies over a lifetime may be necessary to keep returning an individual to this path, and sometimes long-term psychotherapy may supply enough once and for all. I do not see any useful purpose in presupposing, in general, that a great deal of psychotherapy in one block of time is of greater advantage than the same or a lesser amount of time spread out over fifty years.

I am discussing Learning III, in the context of complete therapy, not because it will be achieved very often, but because I believe it gives the most exciting and rewarding life. It is my measure of the most successful work, and so I attempt it whenever the patient aspires to it. Actually, any patient who can be taught to work with his or her own dreams on a daily basis will, ipso facto, be involved in working with the antithesis, unconscious, or shadow opposite to his current thesis or conscious or daytime point of view (see Chapter 13).

Of course, daily practice is necessary but not sufficient, for many patients intellectualize their dreams as a way of resisting their thrust. Guntrip (1968) showed how dreams can be used as a half-in, half-out twilight zone, to keep dependence at a distance. Many other writers recommend them as a high-brow journey into psyche, art, and mysticism, for turning up pleasant symbols.

Relinquishment

The use of the unconscious to overturn the smug piety of the conscious is a rough business. It is what Faulkner (1942/1986) called relinquishment, in which we part from the known for the unknown.

A Case of a Hunter in Dreams

A friend of mine, who is pretty good at relinquishment, might serve here as an illustration of what a hunter in dreams has to cope with. My friend told me of a pair of dreams from one night, which occurred after he made a major discovery in his work. In the first, while his daughter watched, he drew a huge, dark bird out of the sky, beside a river, into a cage without a top. This was marvelous, as if a great power was flowing into him.

In the second dream later in the same night, he was striding into a lecture hall of five hundred people to give a lecture on a subject he had not studied for fifteen years. He was entirely unprepared. The situation got worse and worse, until he was turned out the door, like somebody ill-clothed and held in contempt.

This is a typical sequence, which is hardly ever mentioned by those who would make dreams easy. If he is filled with enthusiasm from the first dream, he is thrown against the wall in the second. He was very relieved to pull himself up out of this second, chastening dream, which played very rough with him for being excited with himself.

I do not think there is any way around this for my patients who want to keep going toward discovery. New and free powers are expansive, so they are always too much for us. If it is sometimes delightful to get them, it is never for long, because they go too far and we have to take a beating to check ourselves.

INCOMPLETE PSYCHOTHERAPY

Hardly anyone is willing to wrestle with his unconscious like this on a daily basis. It is already a big thing to depart periodically from one's prevailing character and get a little free of its drift. Most of my brief psychotherapy is about Learning II. Many patients cannot get free of their driven character without a plunge into the abyss (of the basis fault). They find a little humor in it, or a break here and there, which is Learning I.

Given that the overwhelming majority of patients will be tied to their prevailing story, the best I can do for them is to map where it is going to get a grip on them, and where is the realm of some freedom, and then undergo some passages with them so they learn to make the transition themselves more readily. In classical and religious terms, this is the transition from hell to heaven. The point is to spend less time in hell, but we cannot keep from falling there altogether.

We conclude a passage, and end loosely, knowing there will be more. I do not want it to befall them unawares. That just means that it will take longer to get oriented. Someone who knows his weakness will catch it sooner.

Intellectual knowledge is helpful, but knowledge in words is stronger if it is felt in many different channels, such as pictorially, emotionally, and bodily. I thereby have more chances of noticing that I am getting off course, and so I correct sooner.

This is why I conclude an episode with a patient in such a way as to leave as strong a mapping of the passage as possible, in the sense that mapping is a verbal, pictorial, emotional, and bodily event. This is what religion is all about.

> Memory systems were already naturalized in classical and theological tradition. Basically, these were mental maps, fixed in imagination, on which the whole summa of knowledge and speculation could be arranged, with each item anchored to its place on the map by a mnemonic visual image. *Usually the map took the form of a stairway from the lower Hell, through the intermediate worlds, to the Divine Source.* St. Thomas Aquinas had authorized devices of this kind, partly through the prodigious example of his own colossal memory, and partly through his dispensation (later annulled by Puritans): "Man cannot understand without images." (Hughes, 1992, p. 20; my italics)

Of course, a common Catholic world allowed a common stairway that reached its culmination in Dante's *Divine Comedy.*

> He [Aquinas] was regarded as the patron saint of memory maps of the Catholic spiritual cosmology, and Francis Yates (1966) suggested that Dante's *Commedia* is virtually a memory map of the Inferno, Purgatorio and Paradiso furnished with a sequence of charged images, historically defined figures and self-evident, graphic episodes which become the mnemonic symbols, and the lexicon, of the poet's vision, encompassing his entire intellectual and spiritual universe. The whole work serves as a complete Catholic meditation, formulated like a liturgy, raising Dante (or the reader) from a commonplace, profane condition (the worldly fear of the call) to ecstatic contemplation of the divine source. (Hughes, 1992 p. 20)

I am trying to do something like this, if much more modest, for patients on an individual basis, who live in quite different worlds from the one Catholic world (Mary Smith, personal communication). That world splintered apart.

Let us look then at a few loosely held endings with patients, and the various kinds of memory maps I tried to leave them with.

LEAVING PATIENTS WITH MEMORY MAPS

I prefer to pose back to the patient his very own memory map (Yates, 1966) from his own dreams. If I cannot get him to look in that dark direction, I will make one for him in broad daylight.

A Case of Raging Bull, Revisited

I encouraged this man in the grip of the raging bull to discover a much sweeter side of himself in nature. He became a gardener, who pulled back out of the world and eased up in his pastoral world. We agreed to conclude with such a successful passage.

Just as soon as we agreed to a few more visits, he came in shamedfaced. He had been screaming at his wife again, and she was nearly out the door. She came in the next week to tell me he was two different people, and the screaming one was the one that she was not going to live with. She ended by saying to me that I must not now end with her husband.

I agreed with her. He and I had obviously underestimated his weakness for

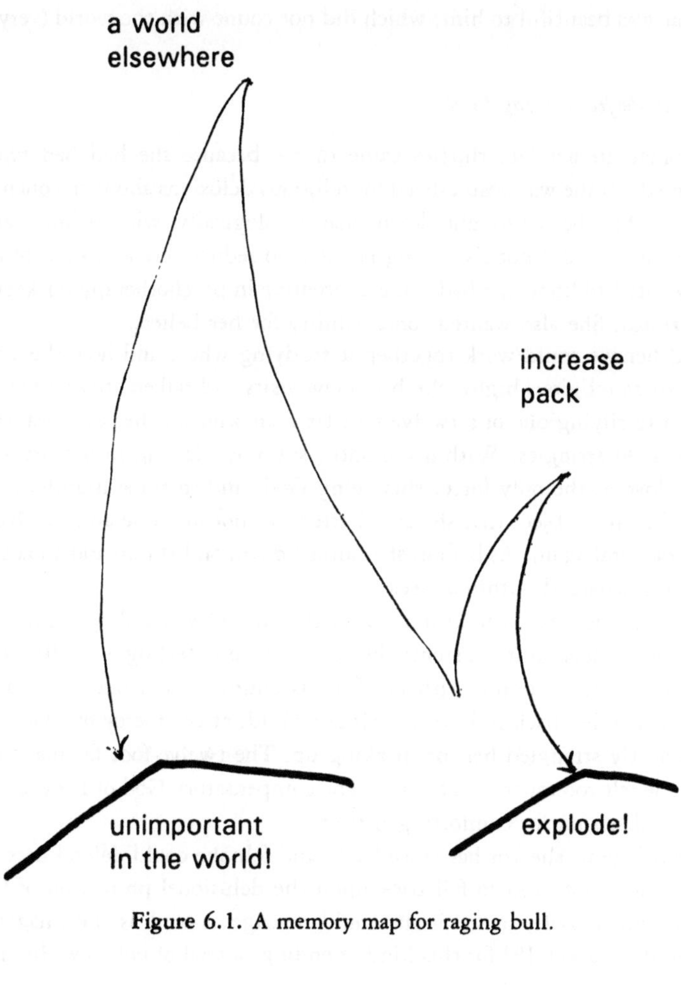

Figure 6.1. A memory map for raging bull.

falling back. Just because we had found a better side that was getting more influential did not mean that the old proclivity had disappeared.

I posed a different ending, with a memory map showing where the increase pack gets ahold of him and stretches him out until he erupts. I told him, point blank, that he would always be vulnerable to this, like an alcoholic to alcohol. If he wanted to keep a family, he had to consider himself flawed and play accordingly. We ended a second time, with his scaling back from many dangerous obligations.

Of course, this made him feel less important, so he was threatened by the prospect of too little accomplishment. This could make him feel like the worthless kid of his childhood, at the mercy of his big, immigrant, hard-driving father.

Indeed, it would be an ongoing dilemma. This was precisely the memory map I left him with. On the one horn was increasing, to feel important, and stretching, until he lost it, which usually happened at home. On the other horn was easing to follow what was beautiful to him, which did not count with the world (very much).

A Case of a Perfect Saving God

A woman in her late thirties came to me because she had had two manic episodes in which she was hospitalized for religious delusions about the oneness of all creation. She had been brought down pharmacologically, with lithium and antipsychotics, but she did not like being handled so reductively as a kind of religious nut. She wanted to know if I had some alternative in psychotherapy for keeping her out of craziness. She also wanted some validity for her beliefs.

I told her we could work together at studying where and how she was transported by these religious highs. We had a few visits and talked about a few dreams, including a terrifying one of a twelve-foot fat man who saw her as a beautiful blue spirit with gold spangles. Within a month, she was slipping into more and more talk about love as the only force, this being God, and in three months she was so obsessed with this subject that she could attend to nothing else and so I had to put her in the hospital again. As before, she calmed down on lithium and an antipsychotic and was discharged within a week.

We spent the next year in long brief therapy, of visits about once a month, clarifying her vulnerability. Essentially, she had been feeling in exile because of leaving her husband, coping with her furious children, and managing a difficult boss. This threw her back to how she felt as a child, at the mercy of a violent father who once nearly strangled her for speaking up. The twelve-foot fat man, in short, got her if she felt too much on her own. The compensatory God of Perfect Love then became her obsession for comforting herself.

Over this year, she got her voice back, and felt she could defend herself pretty well, and would not need to fall back upon the delusional protection of God. We decided to end, loosely, to see if she could manage as well as she imagined. (See Malan [1979, Chapter 18] for this kind of ending, a trial of potency.) Interruptions

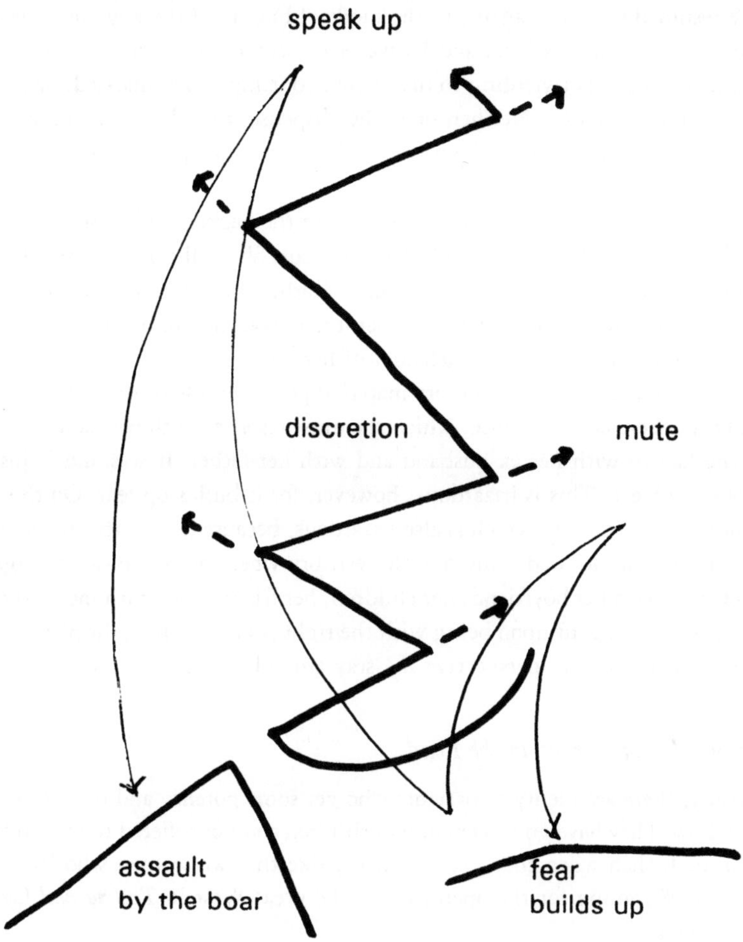

Figure 6.2. A memory map for The Case of a Perfect Saving God.

of treatment of any kind, for a test of potency or for a vacation of the patient or doctor, operate in this way as tests of the ability to bear separation. Malan discusses several variants of interruption, some highly dramatic.

Within two to three months, just as before, she devolved until feeling unduly alone, and the obsession with the God of Perfect Love began to come back. This time we caught it a little faster and got her on a milligram of lorazepam (a minor antianxiety agent that can calm hypomania). She settled down without having to go into the hospital. Just as before, the dream material mapped exactly what happened when she felt abandoned. She dreamt she was holding open the jaws of a Doberman. A doctor said to her menacingly, "No one can hear you. I am going to put you into the hospital." She was back into feeling at the mercy of a devil-doctor-father when I had let her go off on her own.

We resumed our work again, in the mode of long brief therapy once a month. We have had about six sessions, and I have never seen her so strong. She has a new boyfriend, but she is not yielding to his intense courting to get married. She enjoys him and her own house. Neither does she dispense with him just because her children prefer to keep her to themselves. She is her own person, with myself as backing.

I am convinced that I have to stay around in the background to some extent. I do not plan to end at all, but we might lengthen out. She will always be at the mercy of this devil-doctor-father if she cannot locate a father-protector. You just don't ever get over a vulnerability like hers. Rather than have her resort to a delusional protector, I will stay around as a defender of her voice.

She has got a pretty good memory map that poses her dilemmas back to her. On the one horn, there is being mute, which she must resort to with her dangerous boss just as she had to with her ex-husband and with her father. It was and is just too dangerous to object. This is hazardous, however, for it builds up fear. On the other horn, there is speaking up, which is also hazardous, because it risks the direct assault of the boar. She has located some middle territory where her voice can be vigorous and respected, with her boyfriend, her children, her friends, and with me, and this is excellent, but contingent upon being with the right people in the right places. All of this she seems to keep in perspective if I stay around, not too far away.

A Case of Thelma Taking to the Road

Finally, there are plenty of patients who get some potency and do not need me at their elbow. They have gotten enough as children and not suffered too much harm. They can be foolish when they get confident, like the two women who leave their husbands in Wyoming for the open road of the great West in *Thelma and Louise* (a current movie).

I worked with such a Thelma, who was very pleased about divorcing her reliable but restricted husband. She looked forward to finding a more exciting mate with a vitality like her own. It was obvious she stood well upon her own powers as a professional. Unlike the previous patient, she didn't have to have somebody along. She already had a protective parent inside herself. We drew this out, so she could depend upon her own unconscious to read what was coming at her. Indeed, it warned ever so clearly that it was a blunder to climb up the fire tower of a new boyfriend who was ham-handed at pulling her into his aerial nest.

In ten sessions this sort of work got her feeling like she was a pretty good match for the world, with her previous conscious acuity supplemented by this new power to read shadows with her unconscious acuity. She wanted to go on her own, and had a dream as we ended loosely. This was a very precise memory map of the transition between heaven and hell. It was not a stairway, as for Aquinas, but something altogether sudden.

She dreamt she was riding the great highway of the West when she came to a stop. A van backed up right into her face, just stopping short, but right in her face in the windshield. She had two opposing feelings. One was that she was not afraid, because the man driver knew exactly what he was doing. The second feeling was in shadow, but came out in her association about such big trucks.

She recalled a movie in which Dennis Weaver was waved to pass a truck by a smiling truck driver, who also seemed to know exactly what he was doing, but who was waving Weaver ahead to his death. The feeling was fear, and the dream warned her of her excessive trust. She had better look for herself rather than let somebody else read the road for her.

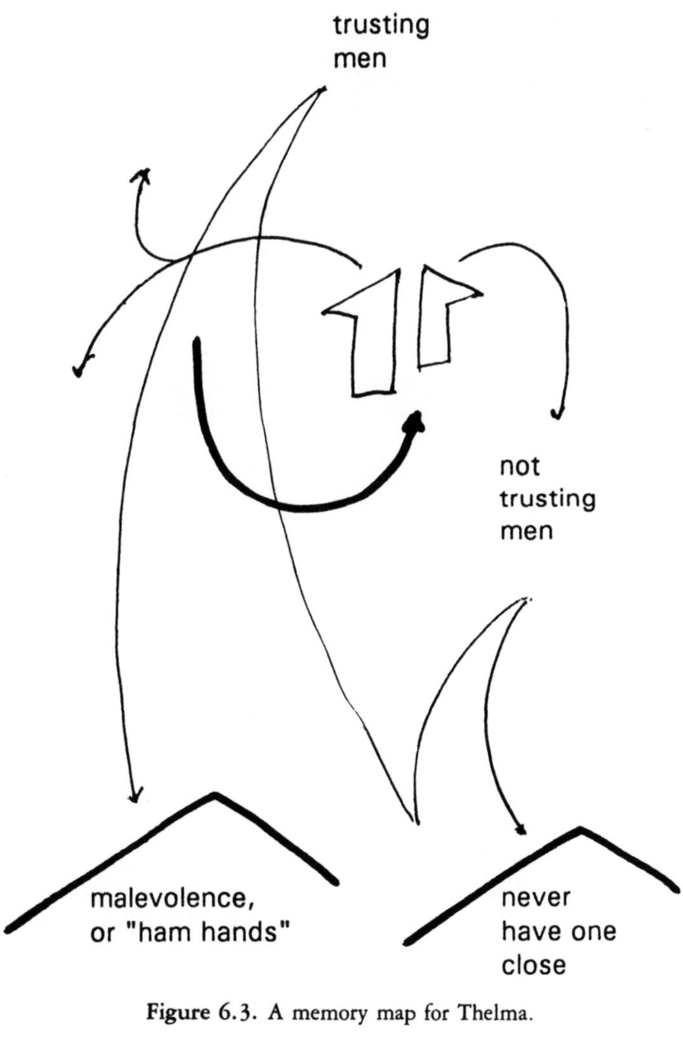

Figure 6.3. A memory map for Thelma.

Here was a very precise and individual memory map of her dilemma of being on a new road of her own expansiveness: On the one horn, there is the need to let powerful men, who seem to know exactly what they are doing, come close, if she wants one for herself. On the other horn, there is the need to feel fear of men who know exactly what they are doing, if she wants to keep from getting knocked off by malevolence. She summarized this pictorial map with the unforgettable phrase of Willy Loman in Arthur Miller's *Death of a Salesman*: "Attention must be paid."

Part II

Simple and Complex Dilemmas

Sailing directions,
landmarks, perils, I shall sketch for you to keep you
from being caught by land or water
in some black sack of trouble
HOMER, The Odyssey

I like to be rudely mechanical about the cars we are asked to fix. Cars have a physics, which we cannot ignore without making them run worse, and so have the plots of stories. *Plot* is an interesting Anglo-Saxon word whose meaning has evolved from a patch of ground, a flat surface, to the ground plan of a building, to design in general, and, most modernly, to a nefarious design (Weekley, 1967, p. 1111). It sounds similar to the word *plight,* which derives from the Anglo-Saxon *pliht*—danger, risk—the verb being *plihtan,* to endanger, later to pledge, promise, especially with troth, referring to marriage (Weekley, p. 1111).

The mechanics of plot and plight concern the dangers built into the design or the promise. Those who ignore the mechanics of the situation go under. Those who purpose to help the patients bound up in these physical plights tend to see their drift into further danger, down the obvious slope of the presenting problem. Their mechanics is applied to reversing the nefarious direction.

This is solution-focused mechanics, and it is somewhat adjusted to the kind of plot that has the patient in its grip. There are three common kinds distinguished by three simple verbs: those who can't, those who won't, and those who must. Those who can't, feeling helpless in their plots of subservience, are empowered by encouragement to believe they can through, for instance, assertiveness training or cognitive behavior therapy. Those who won't, feeling trapped by their own avoidance in plots of delay, are empowered by confrontation that they will get out, but only if they are willing to expose themselves to the danger and go through the terrible phase of anxiety before it is extinguished as, for example, in exposure therapy. Those who must, feeling ruined by their own forcing in plots of overpowering, are empowered, paradoxically, by sharing their helplessness with others so they can be at peace with it and no longer driven, as in Alcoholics Anonymous.

I will illustrate such simplicity of mechanics in Chapters 7, 8, and 9, but I must say at once that solution-focused mechanics are only half right. This is because all problems come in pairs when it comes to plots or plights. If a mechanic reverses a bad direction, the new direction has a slope with its own dangers. The new hazard may be more or less manageable, but a competent mechanic will estimate it carefully. It is what I call the danger on the shadow slope. A common problem in medicine, for example, is how to correct dehydration in an older patient without overloading his cardiac capacity and throwing him into heart failure. In the body, and in the mind, and in these plots, a sound mechanic and doctor will know the alpha error of letting the plot drift further into danger, but also the beta error of turning the plot in a worse direction.

In other words, simple mechanics has to be double to be sound in its application, and this is what I illustrate in Chapters 7, 8, and 9. A so-called double description (Bateson, 1979) is not a luxury but an essential, just as it will not do to understand the cholinergic stimulation of the gastrointestinal system without an equal understanding of sympathetic antagonism. This double description is afforded by the concept of dilemma, which provides the coordinates for all three of these simple double plots. An actual mastery of the plot, thus, is measured by a double test of dynamic change (see Chapter 15) concerning each horn or slope of the dilemma. Can the patient find a stairway back from each of these hellish contingencies?

In my first book, *The Complex Secret of Brief Psychotherapy* (1986), I noted that patients were trying to conserve matters of great consequence to themselves on the inner surface (the surface studied by psychoanalysis), on the outer crust of the inner surface called character (the surface taken up in later psychoanalysis), on the transitional surface between themselves and others (the surface studied by the interpersonal schools), and on the outer surface of objective social structures like families and work hierarchies (the surface studied by the systemic schools). My book showed the triumphs of psychotherapy on different surfaces, from Freud to Reich to Sullivan to Selvini-Palazzoli.

I proposed that there must be a way that this extraordinary evolution of the field of psychotherapy in the last hundred years from inner to outer surfaces might be understood as one rich and mighty subject, rather than as departmentalized disciplines unable to talk with each other because they are looking at different slices of life. Obviously, they were all right on their own surface. But because they ignored the findings on the surfaces that they deemed unworthy of their attention, they all had grave weaknesses.

How were these different levels of description to be put together in a relatively simple way that could be used in a practical way? At the time, I really did not know, and no one did, as Bateson (1979) argued:

> Every evolutionary step is an addition of information to an already existing system. Because this is so, the combinations, harmonies and discords between successive pieces and layers of information will present many problems of survival and determine many directions of change. . . . But, as of 1979, there is not a conventional method of describing such a tangle. (pp. 20–21)

Essentially, I could state the scientific problem without being able to give an adequate reply:

> The difficulty which Bateson discussed at the end of *Mind and Nature* (1979) is that any subject can only be comprehended when it is mapped onto something more complex than itself. "No, you see it's not possible to map beauty-and-ugliness onto a flat piece of paper. Oh yes, a drawing may be beautiful and on flat paper but that's not what I am talking about. The question is onto what surface shall a *theory* of aesthetics be mapped." (Gustafson, 1986, p. 212)

In general, the adequate surface has one more dimension ($n + 1$) than the subject studied (n). Thus, I have utilized in my simple mechanics a surface of two dimensions (dilemma) to map an ostensible problem in one dimension.

The complexity comes from the fact that there are surely four or five valid surfaces on which a patient lives, from the inside to the outside of his life, not to mention all the relevant or salient dimensions on those separate surfaces that are crucial to his well-being. In my second book, *The Modern Contest* (1990, with Lowell Cooper), I distinguished solitude, play, civility, contest, and war, proceeding from the more protected to the most exposed surfaces where we need some measure of control. Obviously, psychoanalysis, character analysis, interpersonal, and systemic work were all directed at extremely important variables on surfaces that none of us could afford to neglect.

I lacked, and we all lacked, a way to move across this incredibly rich terrain with any theoretical economy. The descriptions obliged us to take too much conceptual baggage. We all do it every day, in our practical lives, more or less well. I knew there was an adequate theoretical answer to match the performance that is eminently practical.

The trouble theoretically was that the concepts for describing key structures on any of these fields of observation could not travel over the boundary into the adjacent fields of observation. Thus, psychoanalysts talked about core conflicts, but this was useless in the struggles between people. Character analysis (Reich, 1933/1949) said the constant attitude or posture of the body, the rigidity of the boundary between inner and outer worlds, was the red thread to get us through everything, but it didn't do much for surviving in difficult families. Interpersonal work talked about security operations among our fellows that were closeting, but this told us nothing about the dread in dreams. Systemic work was acute about tricky family games and even the traps in hierarchies at work, but it grossly underestimated character.

I propose to show that the necessary vehicle that can translate across conflict, character, security operation, and paradox is the concept of dilemma. It turns out, in my practice, that, for a given patient, the dimensions of a particular dilemma are relatively consistent from inner to outer worlds, including those transitional worlds in between. This makes the mapping simple. We can have adequate complexity by looking on the different surfaces or fields of observation for possible tangles. This is my subject in Chapters 10, 11, and 12.

Thus, a patient with a subservient dilemma may be tangled up on the inner surface fearing his expansiveness of greed, and tying himself up there in a knot of guilt, which the analysts would call a severe superego bringing about negative therapeutic reactions (Asch, 1976) to spurts of feeling better. He may have a tangle involving his ability to play, which may be dreadfully serious (Winnicott, 1971a). He may have a tangled, rigid character, which has no other god than the one it has known so well, and so panics at any prospect of loosening up (Reich, 1933/1949). He may have a tangle interpersonally, because his spouse is already trained to come down upon him for some of his best qualities (Haley, 1966). He may have a tangle systemically in being unable to read contradictions that tear people apart in his work organization (Selvini-Palazzoli *et al.*, 1986).

Thus, we conclude Part II with a map in hand that has more dimensions ($n + 1$) than the life that is in jeopardy, while we have a simplicity that derives from knowing that any tangle is a complication of the dilemma in question. In other words, we know what to look for. A case may look simple, but the system may be extremely tricky, as Selvini-Palazzoli (1978) wrote:

> How many times we found ourselves literally routed by, for example, the family of a modest postal clerk, his wife an illiterate, his son the designated patient who had seemed completely deteriorated, only able to marvel, laughing over and over again ("Fantastic, they're really fantastic"), realizing once again that great gamblers do not need academic education. (p. 126)

Conversely, the outer world may be simply ordered if tragic, while the dreams are incredibly rich.

Complexity is not a virtue when it is a dodge of simplicity that happens to be cruel (Orwell, 1946). I watched a colleague conduct a brilliant and moving interview of a ruined middle-aged woman. The interview was right in so many ways. It followed her feeling, mirroring her despair, which the Rogerians and the self-psychologists could only applaud. It challenged the harsh superego that had pinned her down and parentified her as a little girl. It acknowledged her longings for love for herself. It surfaced the core conflict between the harsh superego and her need to be loved. It illustrated over and over how this conflict came out in giving herself forbidden things, and then arranging to be punished. The poor patient enacted the conflict in the transference before our eyes, with considerable intensity, by unconsciously stroking herself and feeling dirty. The doctor brought all of this out with much wit, pathos, and originality of gesture and language. Thus, it was a virtuoso performance. I felt it was quite wrong.

It dealt so richly, but it dodged the plot and its grip on the patient. Probably, this was abetted by theories that point to things like empathy and therapeutic alliance and core conflict, for these were attended to beautifully. But the plot is the thing that catches the patient.

Thus, an empty, somewhat odd and pathetic middle-aged woman going into bars to find love is going to get destroyed. This drift of her position was never taken up. The archetypal life of the pack in such places is relentless. If such a woman had her longings for love that was never there pulled for in the safe place of the interview, she is going to have quite a come down after the interview with no company to continue such a conversation. She will have to be cruel to herself in order to get rid of the longing. So this will be even worse on the shadow slope than in the drift of the bars.

The implications are tragic. Everything else but the double plot is relatively unimportant, I think, for we are hired to help someone do what is possible with her fate. This is why my eye is on the plot, first and foremost, and why I think empathy, therapeutic alliance, and core conflict are important for making a connection, but ought not to usurp the point of interviewing. If this woman is not to turn to the bars, where is she to turn instead? This is her dilemma, and this is the problem I would pose to her. It is a bare double plot, extremely simple, and I would keep it that way.

Thus, I am for complexity only when it is in the plot, as a knot that needs to be patiently untied. In Chapters 10, 11, and 12, I will illustrate which of these plots need long-term psychotherapy, and which plots respond to brief psychotherapy, despite their trickiness.

At the opposite pole from the bare, simple, and tragic plot just discussed are the most vigorous patients who pose very different challenges for us. Full-fledged heroes need their mentors very badly, and often do not know where to look for them, and turn to us. Like Homer's Odysseus of nearly thirty centuries ago, they tend to feel constricted staying quietly at home. This life is dull, even a little depressing, for they only flourish in big battles. They go too far in the battles, overextending, and have a terrible time getting back home.

As Jung (1916/1971a) would say, they suffer a psychic deflation at home on the plane of ordinary reality, and they suffer a psychic inflation on the mythical plane of their adventures. This is the double plot of the ancient hero(ine). We had better know something about getting back and forth between psychic deflation and inflation, or we will be useless to them.

Odysseus gets through the horns of his dilemma between Scylla and Kharybdis only when he can give up six men to Scylla. This deflation is terrible, but it is less terrible than trying to stop and fight her and lose twelve. Once through, he and his men are not to eat the sacred beeves of the god Helios, but this inflation runs away with his men when he is off praying, and they all die for it.

The dilemma of the hero is very ancient (Campbell, 1949), and to be of use we had better know it well. This is a very different matter from the lesser plots. We need to be absolutely clear about differences in plot, and that is the burden of Part II, which we now commence.

Chapter 7

Subserving Others May Be Bad for Me

Subservient people are by far the most common in a practice of psychotherapy, because, lacking power, they appeal most readily to borrow it from us. They have in common a posture of diffidence in relation to some greater power for which they have to beg. They vary in their color, tone, and shape, depending upon the place where they must subserve and be ill-used, and thus go by many different names that show their context or locale.

The first patients in psychotherapy were those of Breuer and Freud (1895/1966) described in *Studies on Hysteria*. They were called hysterics, because their dramatic physical complaints were once thought by doctors to be caused by a wandering *hysterus* or womb. Breuer and Freud showed instead that they were servants of families, usually daughters and wives, who were being crushed by their burdens. Nowadays we call them parentified, or adult children of alcoholics, or single-parent mothers, and so forth.

In the sexual domain, the willingness to be used for the sadistic pleasure of another was called masochism. Nowadays we are more likely to think of it as sexual abuse, which has some secondary gratification. The perversions are perverse, in the sense that what is arousing for one is degrading for the one that subserves the dominant.

In the work domain, the names for servility multiply wildly, because each class or nationality seems to have its own. Thus, a fool can be called an idiot, tomfool, wiseacre, simpleton, Simple Simon, donkey, ass, owl, goose, dolt, booby, imbecile, nincompoop, oaf, lout, blockhead, bonehead, calf, colt, numskull, clod, clodhopper, soft or softy, mooncalf, saphead, gawk, rube, greenhorn, dupe, dunce, ignoramus, lubber, bungler, madman, dotard, driveler, old fogy (from *Roget's Thesaurus*). In Yiddish we have schlmozel, schlemiel, schmendrick, and so on. In the middle and upper-middle classes, we have the helping profession syndrome (Gustafson, 1992; Malan, 1979) of doctors, teachers, ministers, and other idealists giving a great deal and getting little back for their troubles. Often, the best boy or best girl is a complete servant of a faculty (Mehta, 1993). Grown up, he or she continues servitude in academic, military, or business terms.

Thus, status may be low, middle or high, but the subserving of others is the thing in common. Subservers have to be allocentric, or decentered from themselves, to sacrifice their egocentrism on this altar of serving others as the center of their lives.

They come to us when they no longer can keep it up. They complain chiefly of lack of interest, depression, anxiety, panic, and bodily ills. They tend to respond to almost any kind of helpful alliance, for they so lack help for themselves, giving it all away to everyone else. They take to it like water for the thirsty.

Our helpfulness is apt to fade if the subservers keep subserving. They will continue to be deprived in their own worlds. Help that lasts, therefore, has got to address the plot.

THE SIMPLE MECHANICS OF THE PLOT OF SUBSERVIENCE

We mechanics have got to understand the engine of the plot, if we are to fix it or help the patient to fix it himself. I think there are three fundamentals. They are not announced by the patient. On the contrary, they will be left out of her narrative. It is like a musical score with gaps in it. If we know the score, ourselves, we will hear what is deleted by the patient. It is this selective inattention (Gustafson, 1986; Sullivan 1954) that hopelessly locks up the patient, for she has no chance at putting her hands on the mechanism that keeps her going around in circles.

The first gap in the story you hear can be located by listening for the patient's amazement (Gustafson, 1986; Sullivan 1954, 1956). He can scarcely believe that he is so badly used by family, lover, or boss. In other words, he cannot quite believe it, which means he is continually caught unawares and, thus, *defenseless*. On these outer surfaces of his life, he is a sitting duck, or a mark, or whatever you call it in his vicinity, drifting down the slope toward wreckage and ruin.

The second gap in the story you hear can be located by listening for telltale words or bodily signs of huge emotion always set in motion in persons badly used. I mean tears and rage. Usually, it too is covered up. These patients usually blame themselves that they are so upset. At the points in the conversation where the feeling is coming up, they often point to their heads in a kind of unconscious self-accusation with one or two or three fingers, which I call Gustafson's sign (1986, 1990, 1992). I will simply comment that they seem very uncomfortable with what they are feeling or that they seem to blame themselves. Often, they reply by asking how I know this, and I just say I sense it to be so. Usually, they respond by dropping their fingers of self-accusation, and the feeling is let out.

Thus, the gap on the shadow slope is usually pointed to by the patient himself, but not always. If you are kept very far away from the situations that are upsetting, by vagueness or diversions into bodily complaints, the feeling will never surface, and will not be close enough to be pointed to as a gap in the text. If the patient is not so self-blaming, the feeling will show more directly, especially in the eyes getting moist, the corners of the mouth drooping, or the voice quavering. I attend to this by saying that something here is very upsetting.

The third gap in the story you hear concerns the dilemma the patient is in once he acknowledges that his being badly used is not amazing on the plane of reality and that his huge feelings are extremely painful on the shadow plane. What is he to do, after all, with the prospect that this is going to continue indefinitely?

Thus, we have descended into hell with the patient, so our company makes it more bearable. It is still hell, and something huge is missing, unless stairways out of it can be pointed to. This is apt to be the most difficult gap to meet. Even if the patient sees ever so clearly where his family or lover or boss is apt to hurt him, he may not be able to defend himself very well. Even if the patient feels ever so deeply his tears and rage, he may not be able to bring it out to anyone but his doctor. No one else may be willing to hear it. After all, tragedy of this kind is routine. This is why interpretation of what goes wrong is often insufficient. It is true as far as it goes, but fails to pose the gap between the shadow feelings and the drifting fate. The patient is left to ponder this question himself. What, after all, is he to do about this dilemma? We ourselves have to know where to look for the stairways out of such hell. We also have to know when there aren't any, or when the stairs lead only so far and the patient is suddenly swept away by worse currents.

THE FIRST GAP IN THE STORY ON THE OUTER SLOPE OR SURFACE

Subservient people aim to please, for that is how they have made a place for themselves. Thus, they are tuned to the frequencies of pleasure of those they want to keep around. They attend to little else, so everything else catches them by surprise.

Mothers as Victims of Their Children

Single-parent mothers routinely fall victim to their children. Why? They devote themselves single-mindedly, often without a thought for themselves. The offspring remain marvelously egocentric. Why not? They are born that way, coddled that way, and continue that way by being so well attended.

This runs along smoothly, until the age of about thirteen or fourteen, when these princes get a pack to run with and begin staying out all night and so forth. The mothers try to put on the brakes, but there aren't any.

Like Bartleby, of Herman Melville's "Bartleby the Scrivener," the lads reply to any request with "I'd prefer not to." Their mothers threaten, and the lads just shrug. As if to say, "Go right ahead and take away anything you want. I don't care about anything. So it won't make a bit of difference!"

The outrages pile up, as in Melville's story, when they refuse all responsibilities, sleep til noon in their rooms, and proliferate pregnancies, debts, and drugs by the light of the moon.

Sooner or later, authorities beyond the four walls of the house get involved. The first charges are usually truancy, shoplifting, and speeding. They progress from there, to the mass police entertainment (Brodsky, 1988) of robbers and cops. The mothers are called upon to come get their sons out of one jail or another. They promptly do at first, grudgingly later. The possibilities are unlimited but for the laws.

I have had many mothers for patients who were caught up with these sons. They are always amazed by what it is that their boys have pulled off this time. They all underestimate the careers into which their boys are launched. They thus apply—like Bartleby's lawyer—a few sanctions.

It is all too little too late. Often there is little left to do but defend themselves from having further advantage taken of them. Naturally, they are amazed that I would think this the case. Actually, it can be helpful to wake the kid up. Without a home base for his piracy, he may have to contemplate toeing the line for somebody!

The virtue of the amazement now becomes apparent. With it, they fuss and worry and occasionally have a fit. All of this occupies them. Once it is recognized for being a routinely futile operation (Gustafson, 1986; Sullivan 1954, 1956), they are thrown back upon themselves. The feelings can be unbearable: tears, rage, and, especially, loneliness, and self-blame. This is tragic, when the son is the only cause.

This is why I point to the dilemma of such mothers. If they get off the slope of being dragged downhill by the kid, they are then on the shadow slope of their substitute possibilities. When there are none, they find this slope even worse than the other. If we can find something latent there, they do much better.

A Case of Helping as an Existential Project

Doctors, teachers, ministers, social workers, and all other helpful people routinely fall victim to their clients. Privately, it is much the same, with their families and friends and in love. This is what Malan (1979) called "the helping profession syndrome."

All of these work-related misadventures are meet with amazement. Of course, I am not amazed at all, and they often begin to pay better attention at the office to what is going to happen next. They are more recalcitrant about their private lives (Malan, 1976a, 1976b).

Let us see how and why. One kind man learned to defend himself better at school, but continued to complain of his girlfriend. She was like a clam he could pry

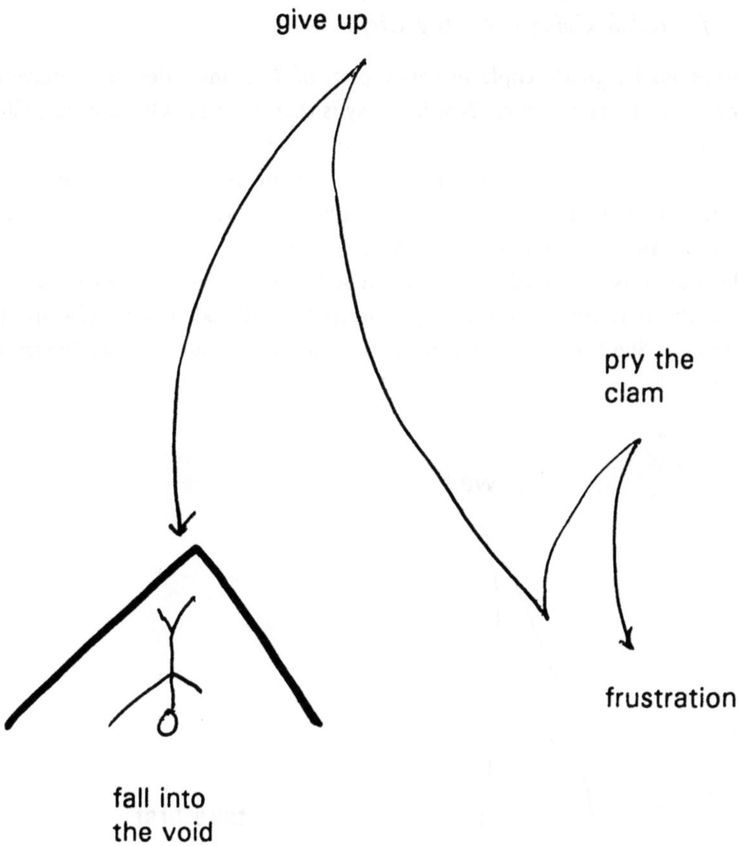

Figure 7.1. A dilemma with a claw.

open a little, but never for long, before she shut tight again at the bottom of her sea. After the best of times, she wouldn't answer her telephone for a week. This went on and on, just like the relationship between John Marcher and Amy Bartram in Henry James's story "The Beast in the Jungle."

I even told him about James's story, because I wanted him to know this could go on for an entire lifetime. He couldn't quite believe it. In our long brief therapy, he reported yet another variation of this same story every month, again and again: A little light when he was about to give up, pulling him back in, then darkness until he would just about lose patience again.

He is still at it two years later, but it makes a little more sense. As long as he keeps poking at it, he has something to occupy his hours away from work. If he were to give up this existential project, he would feel terribly alone in the universe. So it is better to keep it, and its frustration.

A Case of Candide Going to the Big City

Occasionally, good people in this capital of Wisconsin decide to move to big cities for more of an adventure. Not far away is that great brawler of cities, Chicago. But it is not so easy to take a frog out of the pond.

I was quite concerned about this young woman, because every injustice struck as if it were the first she ever saw. Teachers played favorites, bosses were mean, and men took advantage. All were astonishing to her.

She was finishing graduate school in social work, and wanted to see the big world for the first time, after a very protected childhood in a middle-sized town in Wisconsin. She had a job lined up here in Madison, but she was determined to strike out.

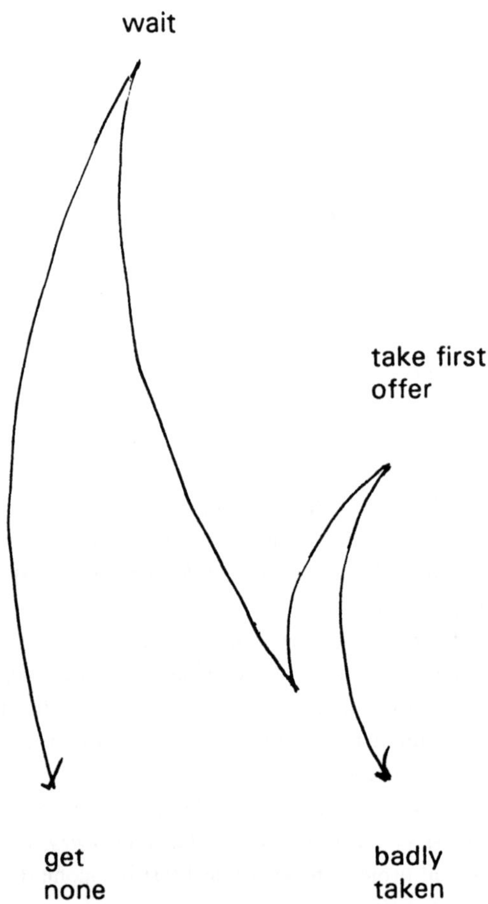

Figure 7.2. Candide's dilemma.

We had ten sessions before she was to leave for Chicago. If ever there was a mark, she was it. Each session was a variation of somebody taking cruel advantage. I would ask what was so surprising? She would tell me she thought people ought to be more fair, more just, more thoughtful. I agreed with her, heartily, because the world would be a great deal better. Since I was no Voltaire's Doctor Pangloss, I did not want to send this Candide to her demise. I told her her plans looked like curtains to me. I was sure she'd be swallowed up her first week in Chicago.

Being a determined young woman, she set about to prove me wrong. She went to Chicago and got several job offers and several lines on apartments and came back to talk it all over with me. She was very inclined to take the first job and the first apartment, even though the job was out of the Loop in a seedy area and she had been scared to death in the hallway of the apartment by the landlord's huge dog. She narrowly escaped by throwing it a sausage and dashing out the front door!

I told her I was very impressed by her bravery, but less by her judgment. Why in the hell was she going to settle for such firsts as came her way? Well, she said, it was better to have something than nothing. I replied that this was an amazing philosophy!

I knew enough about these plots to see the shadow she feared. She was afraid of waiting too long, and thus jumped at the first offer. I told her about the buyer's dilemma, which I invented for her ad hoc. I said that any buyer can indeed wait too long, until everything worth taking is gone, and any buyer can jump at the first and miss what comes along later. She decided that she wanted to be in the middle of the buying, and so desisted.

To my great relief, she figured several sessions later that she was in less danger moving into a place in the city, and taking a job in the Loop, while getting a leave from her present job in case she needed a fall-back position. Now here was an astute woman hedging her bets.

THE SECOND GAP IN THE STORY ON THE SHADOW SLOPE

The subservient car is always a vehicle that comes out of the dangers of childhood. Pleasing key people in your family proves to be less dangerous than angering them, and then it is very serviceable in school. This car breaks down after school, however, on the outer slopes of mating, parenting, and working, where, as we have seen, you are taken advantage of to your perpetual amazement.

Once you challenge this character and call into question its amazement, so that it can see something other than pleasing people, it will be in crisis within itself, because it falls back into its own shadows from childhood, from whence it came (Gustafson, 1986, Chapter 4; Reich, 1949). Thus, the character of subservience is a vehicle that operates outwardly to steer toward pleasing and operates inwardly to put the frights of childhood behind it. Stop the vehicle, by challenge, concerning its outward lights, and you plunge the driver into his particular darkness of the past. This is what Freud and Reich meant by childhood neurosis, which they held must be negotiated in any psychotherapy worth the name. Substitute childhood "vulnerability" and I agree with them. If you are always in flight from it, you are going to drive yourself into a long series of amazing illusions, such as of pleasing people so that they take proper care of you.

Freud's Case of Lucy

In 1895, Breuer and Freud published a report called *Studies on Hysteria,* of their treatment of five cases of subservient women with physical complaints. Two of the women were very disturbed and went on and on with what seemed an endless series of traumatic associations: Anna O. and Frau Emmy von N. One woman, Fraulein Elisabeth von R., had a beautiful result in an analysis of nine months (Gustafson, 1986, Chapter 2); another, Miss Lucy R., in nine weeks; and the last, Katharina, had a momentous single session with Freud on a mountaintop.

The idea that Breuer and Freud had was that these women each had a "single story of suffering" that would be linked by "trains of association" running back from the surface of physical complaints, which would prove to be the "starting points." "The account given by the patient sounds as if it is complete and self-contained." They felt like they were "standing before a wall which shut out every prospect and prevents us from having any idea whether there is anything behind it, and if so, what" (Breuer & Freud, 1895/1966, p. 338).

When they followed whatever associations the patient had to the physical complaint, they reached the "mortification" (Kränkung, or "that which makes ill") which was acting as a "strangulation" of the patient from the inside, or shadow slope. The catharsis of this huge emotion relived the patient from its grip. This had an elegant simplicity like surgery. As Freud (Breuer & Freud, 1895/1966) wrote, "I've often in my own mind compared cathartic psychotherapy with surgical interventions. I have described my treatments as psychotherapeutic operations" (p. 350).

Thus, Lucy, a governess, complaining of the smell of burnt pudding, first associated the smell to the occasion when she got a letter from her mother asking her to return home. She was taking care of the two children of the house, and the forgotten pudding was burned. Freud is shrewd in his guess that she leaves out something about why she must return to her mother, and interposes:

> I cannot think that these are all the reasons for your feelings about the children. I believe that really you are in love with your employer, the Director, though perhaps without being aware of it yourself, and that you have a secret hope of taking their mother's place in actual fact. (p. 155)

The patient admits this "in her usual laconic fashion," explaining that she didn't want to be laughed at. She tells how her hopes were raised when the Director confided in her warmly about how much he depended on her to take care of the children (his wife having died). She waited in vain for a repetition of this intense conversation.

The smell of burnt pudding now faded, to be replaced by the acrid smell of cigar smoke. Here seemed to be a patient with an olfactory mind. She made nothing of this for awhile, Freud insisting and persisting that it would indeed take her somewhere important, and it did. The visiting accountant had kissed the children upon his departure from lunch, only to be shouted at by the Director. "I feel a stab at my heart (notice the present tense); and as the gentlemen are already smoking the cigar-smoke sticks in my memory" (p. 158).

Freud knows there is yet something missing, behind this violent stabbing. There has to be more to it. The final train of association reaches its destination in a scene in which a visiting lady kissed the children on the mouth on her departure. The Director restrained himself in the lady's presence, then burst in fury "upon the head of the unlucky governess, raging and threatening her with dismissal should this happen again. . . . This had happened at a time when she still thought he loved her, and was expecting a repetition of their first friendly talk. The scene had crushed her hopes" (p. 159).

Doctor and patient have reached and relived the single story of suffering, from burnt pudding to cigar smoke to bitter raging, the stench that wrecked her longings, and gave her such huge pain that it strangulated her until it could be brought forth from the shadows. She accepted that she loved the Director, but that her love was an impossible love. A chance meeting four months later shows her entirely well.

A better case of looking for the gap on the shadow slope could not be found. It is true that Freud repudiated this beautiful surgery, arguing by 1905 that the associations had to be taken back further to the childhood vulnerability in a long circuitous journey that becomes the long-term therapy of psychoanalysis, but it is not always so. Like Lucy, many patients are hugely relieved by tracking back from chief complaints into the omitted pain on the shadow slope, and it is quite enough for them. Many patients in brief psychotherapy can link up this pain with the vulnerability of childhood by a simple extension from the present disaster to a similar one in childhood, with wonderful, freeing consequences (Malan, 1976a, 1976b). I will conclude this chapter on simple subservience with just this kind of case, which turns upon a third gap in the story concerning the patient's dilemma.

Before I proceed to the conclusion, I need to add a caveat. About half of the stories of obvious subservience have the underlying dilemma of Lucy. She is harshly injured on the slope of reality because of her having to subserve, while the shadow slope is one of great and excessive longing, which cannot be fulfilled. She seems to be stuck on subserving, but she is equally stuck on her powerful daydreams. These are the two horns of her commonplace dilemma of simple subservience. In every modest life on the surface, look for power in shadow.

Half of these subserving plots have something else in shadow, and that is a tremendous injury to trust from a childhood replete with abandonment and intrusion. In other words, the surface looks like subservience, but the shadow reveals the basic fault.

THE THIRD GAP IN THE STORY OF THE PATIENT'S DILEMMA

I have already illustrated how a primitive dilemma is implicit in subservience stories, where the emphasis of the work falls both on the gap on the outside surface covered by amazement and on the gap on the inside surface filled with unbearable tears and rage. Now, I will show a slightly more complex work whose emphasis falls on the dilemma itself, passing through the amazement and the pain to get to the third element. (Michael Moran, personal communication) in this simple mechanics of subservience:

> Water is H_2O, hydrogen two parts, oxygen one
> but there is also a third thing, that makes it water,
> and nobody knows what that is.
>
> The atom locks up two energies
> but it is the third thing present that makes it an atom.
>
> (Lawrence, 1902/1982)

A Case of Basilar Artery Migraine

A young lady in the university here was referred to me by her university neurologist, who disbelieved a diagnosis of "basilar artery migraine" made by a neurologist in New York City where the patient grew up. Evidently, the patient had had five spells of "lightheadedness, spaciness, fear, and paranoia" lasting five to thirty-two days per episode on five holidays since her junior year in high school.

The neurologist in New York City explained these episodes as a rare form of migraine caused by spasm of the basilar artery at the base of the brain. He gave her a corticosteroid injection during the last episode in an attempt to relieve the so-called spasm. Thus, the patient was heading down a medical slope toward a career of physical illness that could be quite debilitating. She was already failing several courses and in danger of flunking out of the university.

My colleague, the university neurologist, doubted the physical diagnosis because there could be no neurological disorder that brought about spells only on holidays! The link had to be symbolic or situational in the family at that time of year. I suppose it is conceivable that some toxic substance was secreted by their Christmas tree, but this seemed pretty farfetched.

After a preliminary interview in which I found her to be very soundly connected to her parents, to be free of any major psychiatric disorder, and to be thoroughly studied from the medical-neurological perspective, I proceeded to a two-hour conversation with her about the mysterious complaint of these spells, which made about as much sense as Lucy's hallucinations of burnt pudding.

We began with what she was looking for. She, and her parents, wanted an explanation of the spells. I asked her to tell me about how they began. She told me that they began when she was at home on Christmas break during her junior year in high school, when she felt "light-headed, spacy, paranoid, and scared."

I startled her by saying that this was always a distraction. This amazed her, and she looked at me wide-eyed and open-mouthed and asked me what I meant? I replied that these physical sensations were indeed powerful, but they would distract everyone unless understood as a sign that something was bothering her. Still amazed, as in a kind of trance, she questioned me about what could have been bothering her? I simply asked her what came to mind, following the line of questioning so beautifully demonstrated by Breuer and Freud.

Well, she could have been upset that Christmas by her big sister. How so? Well, her sister always got A's, while the patient was lucky to get C's. She might have been resenting having to study so hard that Christmas, while her sister was having it so easy on vacation.

I responded that it sure was a pain having a sister like that. I *know,* she practically shouted, doubling her voice and looking like a lioness. Then, crestfallen, "but my family tells me it is stupid to try to beat her." Here she began to cry. We were near the trouble, but she drew back and told me that she could not say more about that time so long ago.

I said that we might instead take a more recent episode and see where that led us. She agreed, and led me into the Easter just past. She related that the spell began the day she was coloring Easter eggs with a friend, and her mother's mother, or grandma, kept barging in with suggestions, as though she were still a little girl, instead of a sophomore in college.

She got impatient and mad, but began to cry and was taken to task by her mother, looking over the scene in the kitchen. "Why do you always cry?" That night, she woke up in one of her spells.

I asked her about her anger, and it was this. Her mother could yell at her grandmother, but she, the daughter, had to be respectful. Her feeling came out in tears, and that was not all right either, so she just tuned out into her distracting physical sensations! This I summarized for her. That, she said firmly and quietly, hits the nail on the head. We concluded the first hour, and took a little break.

I began the second hour by posing what to me was her dilemma. I told her that trying to deep-six her feelings led to these spells, but owning them might be even worse. Indeed, she feared so. She feared really hurting her grandma, her mother, and her sister! I summarized again, "It seems there is no way for you to own your own feelings without hurting them with your anger."

This put her into contemplation, from which she emerged with an independent discovery (Balint, 1971; Gustafson, 1986, Chapter 8). She proposed that her feelings

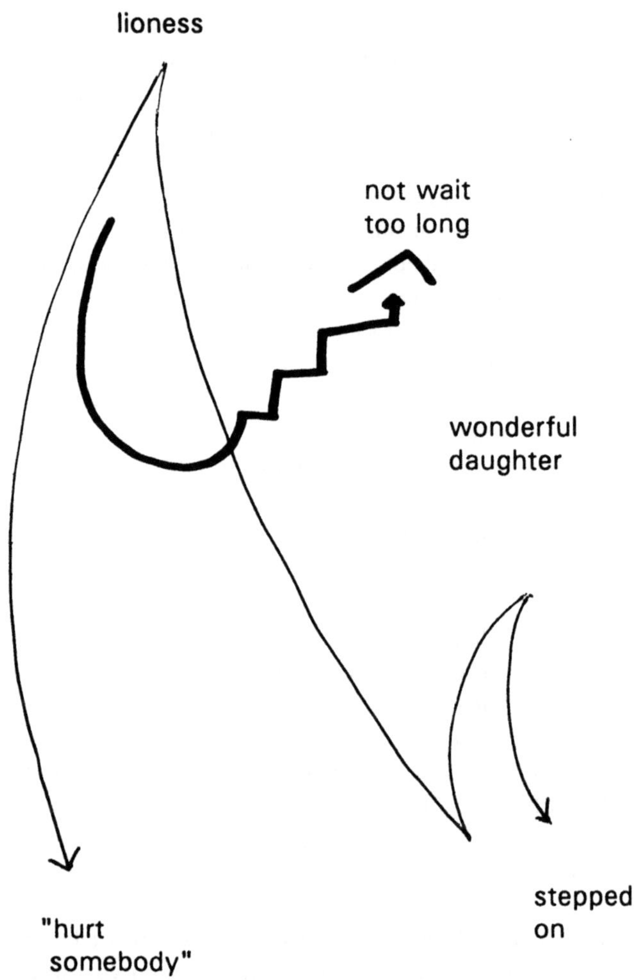

Figure 7.3. A dilemma of a wonderful daughter.

end up hurting other people only because she stores them until they burst out of control. If she spoke up earlier, when they were more manageable, she could be more matter of fact, but then she would not be such a wonderful daughter. She cried softly. She was going to have to give up something, to climb up this stairway out of the hell of being the last in the line of females in the hierarchy of the family. The darling youngest would be less of a darling if she were less subservient.

Thus she reconciled herself, and the episode was mostly solved by this single interview. She had one final question for me. Why didn't the neurologist at home figure this out! She was really mad, and she was going to enjoy telling him off! She laughed with great relish. She was back to being the lioness.

She decided to spend some more time on her dilemma in the family, and did so in ten sessions with a resident, with excellent results (described in the two-year follow-up we return to in Chapter 15).

It is all very much a matter of variations on the theme of this dilemma—between being darling and being assertive. This is the third gap in the simple mechanics of subservience that will be left out of the presenting story.

Chapter 8

I Cannot Decide

Unhappiness is a fall from grace. It has very simple mechanics (Bibring, 1953). Whatever the ideal, there is a come down, and that is depressing. The creature is dispirited, demoralized, world-weary. Any loss, defeat, or setback tends to have this effect.

If the feeling about the fall is shared, many of us often bounce back. This is the idea of grieving. We cry and rage that we have lost something, and thereby detach our longings from that particular object or project and attach them elsewhere and thus recover our interest in the world. This is the gist of Mann's (1973) method of brief psychotherapy in twelve sessions. He names the attempt of the patient at an ideal, say, to be a winning athlete, and he names the pain, say, at losing. This sets grieving in motion. The limit of twelve sessions gives a time frame in which giving up can occur. At its conclusion, there is a giving up as well of whatever excessive hopes were laid upon the doctor or the brief psychotherapy itself.

The weakness of this very appealing proposal of help is that so many of us refuse to take it, because we do not want to give up and grieve. In short, we won't. So we just do not decide about the ideal and the actual. This is the simple mechanics of the plot of delay, which is a delay of grief.

You can look at this delay as a virtue or a limitation, and, indeed it is both. As a virtue, it is called persistence. As a limitation, it is called stubbornness. Whatever you call it, it is extremely common. Perhaps the most common presentation to us is of someone who won't finish something, in school, at work, in a relationship. Another very common presentation is someone who has lost out, but won't let go, again, in school, athletics, work, love, or whatever (Freud, 1917/1963). Another common presentation is someone who cannot make up his mind about anything, because he can't let go of either or any possibility.

These different variations of being stuck lead to tension, which leads to bodily complaints, lack of sleep, frustration, and, finally, demoralization. In the end, this business is exhausting. It also makes people anxious because they get in trouble for not coming through. Other people lose patience with them, run them down, and finally drop them. These patients acquire a long list of diagnoses from psychiatry, starting with a mild adjustment disorder, to neurotic depression, anxiety, and panic, and proceeding to major depression, obsessive–compulsive disorder (Gustafson, in press b), and even schizophrenia. As personalities they are called compulsive, passive-aggressive, schizoid, and several others. All of these disorders are the varying consequences of delay. Like subservience, delay has very simple mechanics, which is often missed because the patient leaves a gap in his account to us.

THE FIRST GAP IN THE STORY ON THE OUTER SLOPE OR SURFACE

I suppose depression is the most common presentation in psychiatry, although it is named by patients in their own terms as exhaustion, tiredness, weariness, loss of interest in things, and being demoralized or discouraged. In every case I have ever seen, I find the patient has taken a fall from his higher hopes (Bibring, 1953). Of course, I find depression because I look for it. However, it is often missed, because the patient claims he is dull for no particular reason. He leaves out his letdown, because it is painful to talk about, and no one is the wiser. The presentation is seamless like a wall.

The dull wall always has a gap in it, which I find by starting from the point when the patient felt well. Following the patient along from his wellness, I soon come to his disappointment with the world. It is an extremely simple matter, and yet it is routinely overlooked. The gap turns up by tracking the downward course.

A Case of Depression in the First Week of School

This case stands out in my mind from ten years ago (Gustafson, 1984), because it so vividly illustrates the kind of dull, flat, and uninteresting presentation that turns off doctors from looking further. I remember the patient even dressed in shades of brown, with a listless voice, and no light in her eyes. The resident presented her to me after his preliminary interview.

Essentially, I was told that this young graduate student was depressed for no reason during the first week of school. It was not rational for her to be so. This was someone who wasn't any good at talking anyway. The resident thought that she just needed antidepressants. We have seen hundreds of patients like this.

What was startling about this young woman was her sudden transformations. When I asked when she had felt better, she replied she was just fine the past summer, riding her bicycle all over Indiana. All of a sudden, she was alive again, telling me this, and laughing about her adventures on the road. She had been a free woman, and just telling of it breathed life back into her.

I said to her, let's follow this along and see what hit you. Well, she replied, I was fine for several days, until about mid-week during the first week of school. Oh, I said, tell me about the day you went down. Well, she said, it was in a class in the business school, a class she needed to complete her degree.

"I started to sink, as soon as the old professor began to ramble about the text for the semester. It as an outmoded text, taught by an outmoded professor. The prospect of listening to him for two hours a week for the next twelve weeks was disheartening. It was the collapse of my summer."

Now, she looked blank again, looking for all the world like there was nothing to her. The gap was only apparent by tracking her backwards to where she was really with us, and thus we could find the very place where she went off the road into this ditch of despondency.

From here, the thrust of the interview was not difficult. All I had to do was ask her to tell me about her feelings about people like this wasting her time. Of course, I found her outrage, and her guilt (the latter by Gustafson's sign of pointing in accusation at her own head, following right upon the first show of her anger). Her guilt took us back to her father, who had also enraged her. She had been put down in a cruel way for opposing him. Now she put herself down and collapsed into this depression, when she found herself angry at another old man. Once we knew the place where she went off the road, the direction of the interview was as straightforward as Freud's interview of Lucy (see Chapter 7) from the place she went off the road, which was marked by the smell of burnt pudding.

The difference is that depression tends to cover its own trail with its vague and dreary cloud. Therefore, we just have to know how to back up, like a videotape, and bring the patient back to life so we can see the painful fall.

Many psychiatrists take depression at face value as a biochemical lapse. Of course, depression is accompanied by profound biochemical changes, but I find it is more often triggered by the world than by mysterious medical events. However, hypothyroidism can cause depression, and so can the onset of diabetes, and we must always look for the medical etiologies in every depression (see Chapter 2).

The virtue of psychiatry to look for the medical etiology is also its weakness. Once you get busy with that kind of work-up, you may well have passed by the patient's pertinent history. Simply backing it up, as I have suggested, can bring significant findings out of the gloom. My last five consultations to the affective disorders inpatient service turned up these findings, which had been completely missed: a businessman who worked sixteen hours a day and bought a new house that needed repairs, but could not subtract any time to work on the house from his very long day at the office; a frantic woman who was being cut out of her inheritance by her father's second wife, but could neither fight it nor beg to be let in; a woman coming into middle age was successful at work, but forlorn with no prospect of a husband; a nice old lady who wanted free of the burdens of her four grown-up children, but could not say no to her youngest moving back in along with her penniless husband and two noisy little kids for a two-month visit that became two years; a doctor who gave up overseeing six public clinics to take up private practice, but became swamped by endless business details.

All of these people were depressed to the point of being admitted to the hospital for being suicidal or unable to carry on taking care of business. Some were agitated as well. All became agitated when I drew out the history, because I got them to face the fall that could not be borne. Essentially, they were giving up. All got better in the hospital, simply by getting away from the outside surface of their lives, which was a disaster. Of course, they would have to return to it, and therein lay the unfaced difficulty.

This is the usual sequence. Something grand is attempted. The patient works doubly hard to pull it off but becomes exhausted. This agitates him as he senses his downfall. Finally, he collapses into a blank despair. The businessman, the inheriting lady, the middle-aged lady, the nice old lady, and the doctor all followed the same course.

Once you believe, as all of these people did believe, that you simply ought to push yourself doubly hard when your burdens double, then it is only a matter of time to your downfall. This is the simple mechanics of delay on the outside surface, which refuses to face the limits of what you can make yourself do.

Sometimes the refusal is not so gross. In the outpatient department, I often see a delay that is crippling, but the patient can limp along indefinitely. For example, a young woman who was an excellent student in her little high school comes here and can barely cope with the academics of the big university. Rather than ask for help, she pretends she can manage it all by herself, but has panic attacks at exams. For another example, a middle-aged teacher is wearing himself out with a huge load of students plus a night job. He can keep it going, but he compensates himself by uncontrolled eating in the evenings. The young lady wants to be rid of her panic, and the teacher his mounting obesity, but neither wants to see that she or he is attempting the impossible. The panic and the urge to eat just don't make any sense to them. They are just being rational people, struck by irrational feelings.

These people stay so busy that they do not have to notice that their activity will not get them where they want to go. They are putting off the reckoning, but it will tax them until it takes them down.

It is very important to note that some of these hard workers simply have to continue because it is worse for their souls if they do not exhaust themselves. At least they get a little sense of worth from their efforts. If they do not, they feel worthless. They fall back into an abysmal childhood that was truly unbearable.

A Case of Luther's Dilemma

A man worked himself in his business from dawn to dusk, whereupon he went to bed spent. He complained to me of increasing stiffness. Indeed, he would only become more so because he was either bent over his accounts or he was in bed. Secretly, he loved his bed, which was his only refuge.

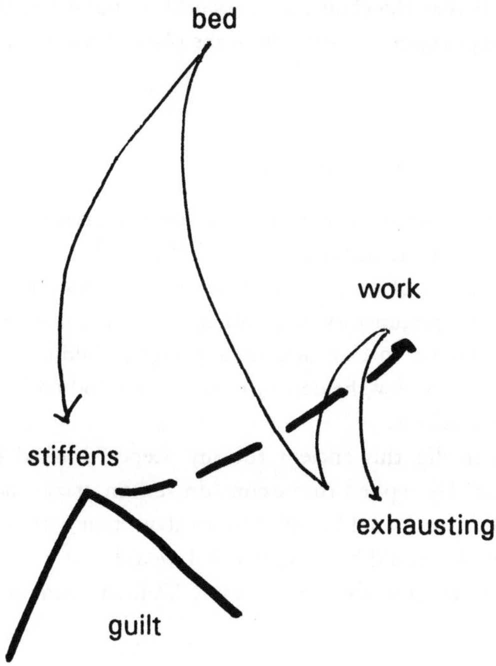

Figure 8.1. Luther's dilemma.

Whenever he tried to take a break from this diurnal routine, he was tormented by doubts about his worth. These doubts resounded in his ears, as if they were from the cruel mouth of his patriarchal father.

He was really better off working, which silenced this father, and then going to bed when he had worked himself long enough. He was amused when I told him that Martin Luther had had a similar dilemma. He did have a little sense of humor, which I could arouse by telling him how terrible it was to be in his situation. So it was a kind of gallows humor. He even made a few reforms in his business association, which was his equivalent to the Catholic Church of Luther.

Many patients who exhaust themselves in the world are like my patient, who dares not let in his shadow side. The shadow slope slides directly into a pit of hell, which is the basic fault.

THE SECOND GAP IN THE STORY ON THE SHADOW SLOPE

The opposite stance to being busy is not to be busy at all, but to daydream like Washington Irving's Rip Van Winkle and wander in the woods with your dog. This activity has the very same effect, wondrously, of postponing the fall from high hopes. Whereas the busy distract themselves from their longings by activity in the world, the avoiders pretend that the claims of the world do not exist. By either method, mythical being is kept rigorously apart from the plane of reality in which the patient has a small part.

A Case of Being Fully at Home in Baseball

I first met this young man when he was being interviewed by a resident who took complete charge of the interview. The resident's idea was to get to know the patient by making a tour of his past. The young man's answers complied with the questions in a sad and perfunctory way. When the young man replied that he had been his mother's deputy, to look after four younger children in the absence of a father, I could see he was now the deputy of the doctor and no happier about it. He postponed his own business.

Not wanting to dig this ancient rut any deeper, I asked him what he was looking for from us. He replied that exams drove him crazy, and he had one this evening! I responded that I would be glad to see about that with him if he liked, and he quickened to say he would be delighted if I would.

I asked him to tell me about this exam. Well, he said, it ought to be easy

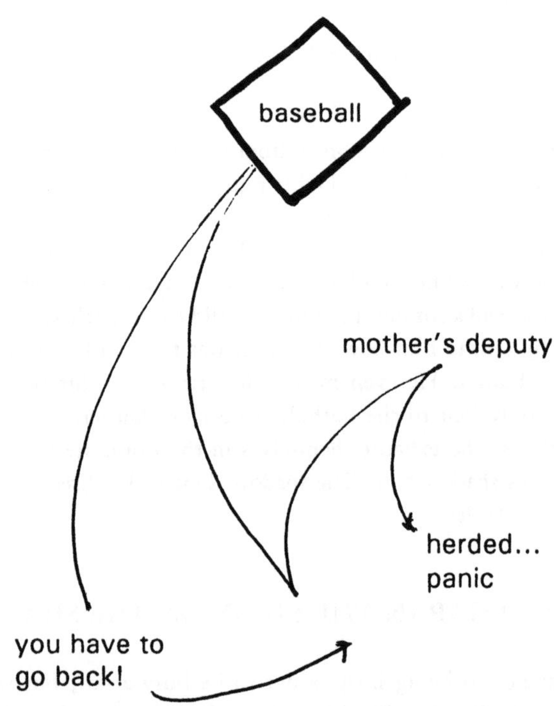

Figure 8.2. The dilemma of being at home in baseball.

because it was multiple choice on an easy subject, but he surely would be shaking when they opened the door to let in the students. He hated it because it was an ordeal. Indeed, he had made it as far as this senior year of college by finding professors who would let him do essays or delay taking exams to when he could be alone with the test. This was how a university ought to be adjusted to the needs of individual students, he explained to me. Herding them into a hall and making them submit all together was very unnatural.

This was a very interesting phrase to my ear, so I asked him what, then, was natural? Rather than holding him to my purposes, I was trying to follow his, and this distinction between unnatural and natural must have been very close to the center of his existence. He answered that in baseball he was completely natural. It came to him effortlessly, and happily. I was moved by his joy, and exclaimed it was his true home. He went on to tell me all about it.

Unfortunately, I noted, you have to take the damned tests. Yes, he said, it's like being forced onto a roller coaster and strapped in for the ride. It makes you sick.

Well, I had found where he lived and where he died, and walked with him from the one place to the other in such a way that I was there for him, and not he for me. I had earned his trust in this little walk, and he was to come back and make use of it (as I will describe in Chapter 15).

Chucks

What I want to point out here is the just-described patient's vital existence in an out-of-the-way place that his professors would never guess, his home in baseball. I had another patient who found it at sea in the merchant marines. Another told me he was a woodchuck. I was explaining the psychology of these men in their separate territories as worlds elsewhere (Poirier, 1966) to an audience in a workshop. They instinctively knew what I meant and told me about sky-chucks and office-chucks and career-chucks and beach-chucks and couch-chucks and even numb-chucks. They live in shadows, often very intently, and appear flat and dull and nondescript to the world.

The trouble is that the world is sooner or later going to press them, flush them, and hound them out of their chucks. That is a very terrible thing.

A Case of Psychosis at Sea

I happened to see this man when I was rounding on our inpatient service, and I invited him to come talk with me and the medical students I was teaching to interview. He had become psychotic at sea, imagining that the officers were out to kill him, so he had attacked the first mate with an axe. Now no longer psychotic, with the help of antipsychotics and six weeks time, he was being evaluated for a defense of not guilty by reason of insanity. From my studies on psychotic decompen-

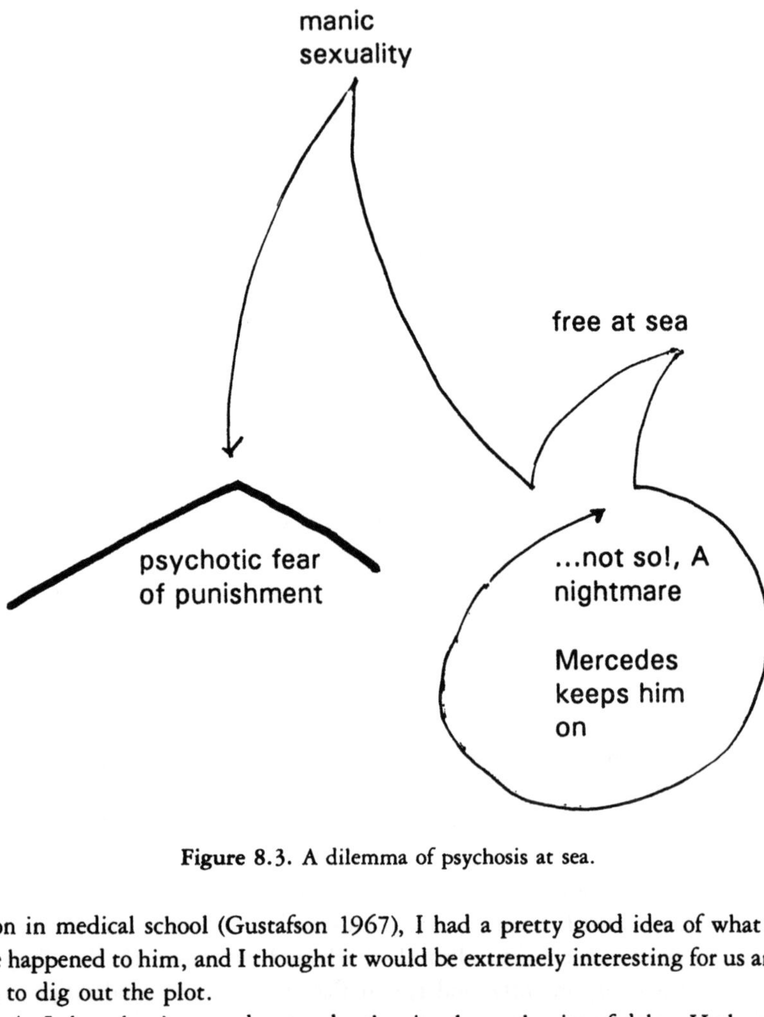

Figure 8.3. A dilemma of psychosis at sea.

sation in medical school (Gustafson 1967), I had a pretty good idea of what must have happened to him, and I thought it would be extremely interesting for us and for him to dig out the plot.

As I thought, it turned out to be the simple mechanics of delay. He loved the serenity of the sea, to him a great relief from the hassles of land. As he put it to us, with childlike charm, you get up in the morning and walk out on deck and it's beautiful and peaceful, and somebody makes you breakfast, and you don't have to fight traffic jams to get to work.

Unfortunately, he got a ship that went north into Arctic waters, where it was dark and cold and completely inhospitable and even terrifying, with the ice bumping the ship's sides in the night. Worse, the company was trying to save money and worked the men seven days a week. Furthermore, his roommate was always drunk, so he had no outlet there. He felt the strain just where he had counted on being peaceable.

Having gotten increasingly depressed, he now flipped into manic sexuality and masturbation, and could hardly sleep at all. Soon he was exhausted. He started to imagine that the officers were going to punish him for his sexual transgressions. He was able to go to the ship's nurse, who listened; the patient cried and was greatly relieved for the time being.

Hoping for a break, he had written relatives in England that his ship was docking in London. This was of no help, as his cousin was cold, menacing, and critical of any little detail, such as his blowing his nose. Back on ship, he began to get more tense.

He overheard a remark of the first mate, as if he were saying that the patient had to be hanged. He barricaded himself in his room, and waited behind the door with the ship's ax. After an agonizing and endless night during which no one came, he went up on deck and went after the first mate. Fortunately, several men were able to disarm him and put him in the brig.

Of course, the patient left the most important part out of the story, which I now asked him about. Why did he not quit the ship, if it was sending him straight down hill in this nightmare? He laughed when I asked him. "Oh that," he said. "I had planned to fix up a very beautiful car, a Mercedes, and I needed the money. So I stayed on!"

Falls from Heaven

So much of the grief in these cases is about colliding with evil in a fall from heaven.

The Simple Mechanics of Delay in Psychosis and Other Kinds of Basic Fault

This is the gist of what I found in my studies twenty-five years ago (Gustafson, 1967). The patient stays in an increasingly untenable situation, trying to hold onto something precious to him. It is an extremely dangerous thing to do, but the patient had nobody to face it with him and finally begins to hallucinate to a god of last resort. At this point, he leaves reality. Then the god turns cruel. So the help hallucinated turns into a torment hallucinated.

I certainly cannot generalize this plot to cover all psychoses, for many are driven by imbalances of neurochemicals, which, in turn, derive from many medical conditions. The just-described patient had both a psychology vulnerable to abandonment and a manic frenzy when depressed. All I can say is that this plot, with its delay, is extremely common in psychosis.

There are many patients who live in shadowy comfort and who cannot take the demands of the world and who resist by means other than psychosis. Many just stay hypochondriacal and oblige doctors to work them up endlessly. Others can't leave the house, and get the diagnosis of agoraphobia. Still others ruminate and ritualize and get the diagnosis of obsessive–compulsive disorder (Gustafson, in press b). These are variations on putting off the world—staying in bed to read detective stories. By and large, this works pretty well, unless the doctor thinks he can force the patient out of her squirrel home, but this is usually futile.

THE THIRD GAP IN THE STORY OF THE PATIENT'S DILEMMA

Some patients try to do the correct thing, and work vigorously to keep up their place in the world. They also have some kind of chuck that is dear to them, and they run to it whenever they can. Living becomes an alternation between obligations and retreats. This plot is slightly more complicated than the plot of unending obligation or the plot of obstinate retreat.

I first encountered it in a fraternity at the Massachusetts Institute of Technology when I was eighteen. The fraternity brothers knocked themselves out for a week, acting like all-American boys, playing every sport imaginable in the sunlight. I was impressed and signed up as a pledge to live there. Friday night, the pledges now signed up, the brothers got horribly drunk and dragged a cohort of women in and acted like gross barbarians.

I was completely dismayed, being completely fooled by the plot, which turned out to be a weekly cycle. Sunday night they would sober up and work like Puritan ministers all week. Friday night they would lapse into their sadistic excesses, mostly directed at women, but also at us pledges, and to some extent at their rivals in the hierarchy of the house. It was truly a day and night turnabout.

I had little idea that this plot was of some general import, so I got out of there and went to Harvard. Thirty-three years later, I call it the German dilemma, defined as follows. The drive to do things correctly is what places you in a hierarchy, of engineers, as at M.I.T., of lawyers, as in political science at Harvard, or of doctors at Harvard Medical School. It always asks too much of you, and you strain to make yourself comply. Later you get a little freedom and you can take it out on somebody else. The plot cycles between a moral masochism (Brenman, 1952) by day, and a moral and sexual sadism by night.

The German Dilemma and Freud's Rat Man

This is an extremely redundant story, and I call it the German dilemma not because it is confined to Germany but because it is so gross and obvious there. The patient was a law student (Freud, 1909/1975) taking exams and about to take on a practice. Indeed, he was offered an opportunity to have an office fixed up for him by a relative of Rubensky. The temptation was to take it, but it would mean giving up his true love, Gisela, whom he could not afford to marry, and marrying one of Rubensky's daughters instead.

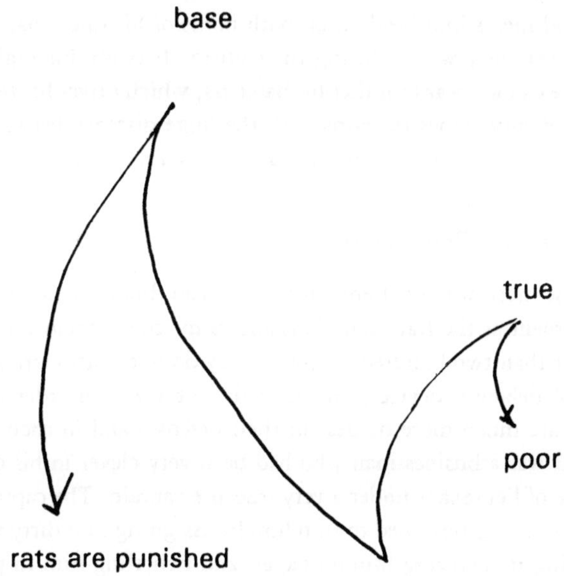

Figure 8.4. The German dilemma of the Rat Man.

The patient then falls into his oscillations between being base and being true. If he is true, he is poor, and that cannot be. If he is base, he is disgusted with himself, and suffers torments of conscience. He goes back and forth ceaselessly, and exhausts himself, until he comes to Freud in a delirium.

The psychoanalysis of this man in eleven months (perhaps five times a week, or about two hundred sessions) is neither brief psychotherapy nor very long psychotherapy by today's standards. (We know it was eleven months, and we know from Freud's [1909] original record of the case that it was to some extent a daily analysis, but his notes are intermittent.) For me, it illustrates why a classic delay can be prolonged beyond the range of a brief psychotherapy, which is usually only twenty sessions or less.

Freud's analysis is fiercely devoted to addressing this man's dilemma with great clarity. First, Freud points unceasingly to the man's attempts at being indefinite, slippery, and obfuscating. The man has an entire catalogue of such operations for pretending that his dilemma over having success and having his lady will go away. It won't.

This conflict agitates the patient and throws him into his ferocious entitlement, which he inflicts on Freud himself, in terms of sadistic fantasies about Freud's own daughter, and so forth. The patient then becomes terrified that Freud is the famous train murderer, Leopold Freud, and will take his revenge upon the patient. Freud is instead kind to him, and clarifies his wild transferential distortions. Sullivan (1956) emphasizes that obsessionals often stay somewhat secure by making others impotent to object. The Rat Man certainly tried this on Freud, without success, because Freud could not be swerved from the Rat Man's dilemma. Freud would not be sidetracked.

Thus, Freud meets him head on on both horns of his dilemma, both impossible. He cannot get away with delaying the collision between his high idea and his low need, and he cannot bear to inflict his baseness, which drives his terror about the revenge. He gradually comes to terms with the huge distance between his entitlement and his actual limiting circumstances, and settles down.

The Case of the French Bullet Train

Fortunately, most of my patients in the German dilemma are not as steeped in Prussian entitlement as the Rat Man. This allows me to see them through its horns in twenty rather than two hundred sessions. They do not resist clarity with such an enormous set of delaying devices, and they do not try to murder me with their baseness. They are much more modest in their defenses and in their claims.

My patient was a businessman who had been very clever in his career until he rose to the place of lieutenant under a very insecure captain. The captain feared him for his cleverness, and determined to ruin him by assigning him dirty work, faulting him for not doing it, harrying him on paper, and belittling him in person as if he were a mere clerk. He was sent to me by his internist, who made his referral when the patient kept getting colds, his diastolic blood pressure went up nearly to one hundred, and it was evident that he would be fired. Naturally, he was demoralized, but his wife, a very fierce lady, kept insisting that he keep fighting. He felt doubly a failure, once for being unable to cope with the captain, and secondarily for being unable to be as sanguine as his wife wanted.

I saw him for thirteen sessions, with excellent results on four-year follow-up (see Chapter 15 for the follow-up). The therapy fell in thirds, in terms of its focus, quite along the lines of this chapter. In the first third, I dealt with his amazement at the cruelty of his captain. My patient was so busy doing the right thing that it never occurred to him that a superior would ever nail him for his virtue. He had prided himself on staying out of harm's way. I especially remember him describing how he stole out of gym class to the balcony to skirt the teasing in the showers and how he coached third base in softball so he never came to bat. His selective inattention missed the dangers from authority, so busy was he looking out for peers. He assumed that the authorities liked smart kids, so the attack came upon him blind-sided.

In the second third of the therapy, I dwelt upon his feelings at this grave injustice to a fine man. He did not allow them easily, abetted by the stoicism of his wife, who did not approve of his tears and rage at all. I did. I recall even backing his showing his young son the cows at the university farms every morning on the way to work and every evening on the way home. The patient then asked me if he could have one of my fine Chesapeake cookies! and told me a most marvelous dream that bespoke his dilemma. This was the seventh and pivotal session.

In the dream, he is riding a French bullet train across Canada, from west to east, backwards, as it were. It is a perfect system, only it had to travel through two

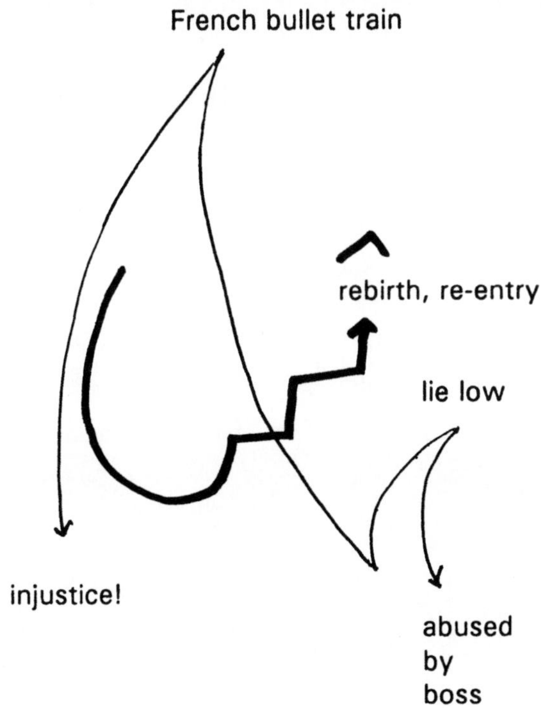

Figure 8.5. The dilemma of the French bullet train.

ice tunnels. When it reached the east (Toronto), it was washed off, purified, and returned west.

In his associations, the French bullet train is his idol, the perfect system to save him from all harm. It lives, like his son's cows, and it is his love. Yet he has to live out the summer in his office before being transferred back to an old office of lesser repute, and this feels cold and dirty, as in the ice tunnels and as in the dirtying of the beautiful train. Here he was near tears, in the poignancy of his own plight, but not for long. The train was washed, as he was with me, purified, and returned west to face the world bright-eyed again.

This beautiful dream literally travels between his perfect ideal and system and the cold and dirty degradation suffered in this world. It returns holding onto the ideal and the actual in excellent humor. We spent five more sessions on his outrage.

[illegible]

[illegible] was washed off, purified, and [illegible]

In the dream, the French bullet train is his idol, the perfect system to save him from all harm. It lives, like his son's cows, and it is his love. Yet he has to live out the summer in his office before being transferred back to an old office of lesser repute, and this feels cold and dirty, as in the dark tunnels and as in the dirtying of the beautiful train. Here he was near tears, in the poignancy of his own plight, but not for long. The train was washed, as he was with me, purified, and returned ever to face the world bright-eyed again.

This beautiful dream literally travels between his perfect ideal and system and the cold and dirty degradation suffered in this world. It returns holding onto the ideal and the actual in excellent humor. We spent five more sessions on his outrage.

Chapter 9

I Am Entitled

We are an extremely expansive species. When we have staked out territory A, we eye the neighboring territory B, and soon we attempt to impose the same horticulture, or armament, or business. We lack modesty and measure. This is evident from Bosnia to Palestine to South Africa, or from New York to West Berlin to Peking—that is, north to south, and west to east.

Not all of us are so openly acquisitive, so we exist as *formes frustes* and vicarious participants in the violence and sexual mating that are the chief and continuous subjects of planetary television: that is, mass police entertainment (Brodsky, 1988). Those who openly display their vitality and greed are followed avidly by those of us who subserve them, or delay our own big ideas. This dominant third knows, as Merrill-Lynch suggests, no boundaries. This is the very simple mechanics of entitlement, that is, to cross boundaries willy-nilly, an act that is essentially overpowering.

Entitlement is smiling when it is having its way. When it reaches an obstacle, it turns dark and wrathful and becomes the she-wolf, the lion, or the leopard. In Dante's *Inferno,* these are the symbols, respectively, of incontinence, violence, and fraud, in descending order from horrible, to more horrible, to most horrible.

In modern and psychiatric terms, we call these plots and their personalities narcissistic, cyclothymic, borderline, antisocial, sadistic, and paranoid. They do not like to see us—an admission of weakness. But they come, under compunction and threat. We see them a great deal when the people they are driving crazy can appeal to us, when they have to come along, as in marital and family therapy, and in emergency rooms where they alarm doctors, or in prisons where they are finally contained. I see them in individual psychotherapy, brief and long, when forcing things has hit a wall.

THE SIMPLE MECHANICS OF THE PLOT OF OVERPOWERING

Entitlement, being so charming, is pleased with itself. We are won over, until it finds a limit and turns dark. This is very important to understand if we are to be ready for the suddenness of the overpowering. I think the medieval minds were much clearer about this than we are now, in their conception of the devil himself:

> And so Augustine, in the book *On Free Choice,* assigns the devil's sin to the fact that he delighted in his own power, and in *Commentary on Genesis 4* Augustine says that if the angelic nature turned to itself, often the angel would take more delight than in that by whose participation it is blessed, and swelling with pride, would fall. (Aquinas, 1972, p. 78)

This is the plot of overpowering in its simplest form: self-delight, swelling with pride, the fall, and violence.

THE FIRST GAP IN THE STORY ON THE OUTER SLOPE OR SURFACE

The simplest way to say what is true about us when we feel entitled is that we expect to have our way. Because we have had our way, we expect to have it again. In other words, we presume, and miss the evidence that our claim will be seen as invalid. We are amazed and shocked to be brought up short.

A Case of a Prophet in the Temple

I could have saved this man a lot of trouble twenty years ago if I had understood then what I am saying now. Being gifted, he did not distinguish well between creating things and showing them. He ran from the first into the second, as young and excited people do regularly.

The Department of Psychiatry at that time used to be called the Temple, ironically by some and quite literally by others. This young resident was very pleased with this idea, and liked as well to think of himself teaching there and overthrowing the pharisees who dominated the upper floors. Indeed, he was a very interesting student to listen to in seminars.

What caught him completely by surprise was that he was stepping on the toes of faculty who preferred to pontificate themselves. He did not know his place. After two years, they decided to teach him a lesson, which laid him flat. They summoned him to a review, and told him he'd have to take over much of the second year and be subject to examinations to boot.

This is what brought him down, extremely hard, and brought him to me as a patient. Naturally, he was full of tears and rage, which came out readily. He was also depressed, because he could no longer uphold the grand picture of himself as a prophet. But he was resilient and did not stay down for long.

Soon I was hearing about his dreams of revenge. This was quite a series of dreams, but I remember now but two, which being so striking have stayed with me. One was of him as a commodore sailing an old frigate down the halls of the upper floor of the Temple, pausing at each door, and letting go of a fusillade of cannon balls until he had finished off the entire faculty. A second was of him sitting astride the tail of a 747 jet, and flying right down the canyon of Wall Street, with some devastating effect I cannot now recall.

At the time I only heard him out, which was cathartic for him. If I had known better, I would have taken up the psychic inflation (Jung, 1971) so obvious in these two dreams. Obviously, he is not the commander of a frigate that is much too big to sail down the halls of the Temple, and obviously he is not the tail-commander of a 747 that is much too big to roar down Wall Street. The dreams call out the very absurdity of his claims.

The gap in his story is quite evident on the outer surface of activity within the department. He presumes to teach, when he is but a beginner, as if the faculty would be glad of his creation, as if he could just transpose the creations in his own mind onto the field of faculty dominance. Thus, he was completely unprepared for their retaliation.

With what I have learned in twenty years, were he my patient now I would hear

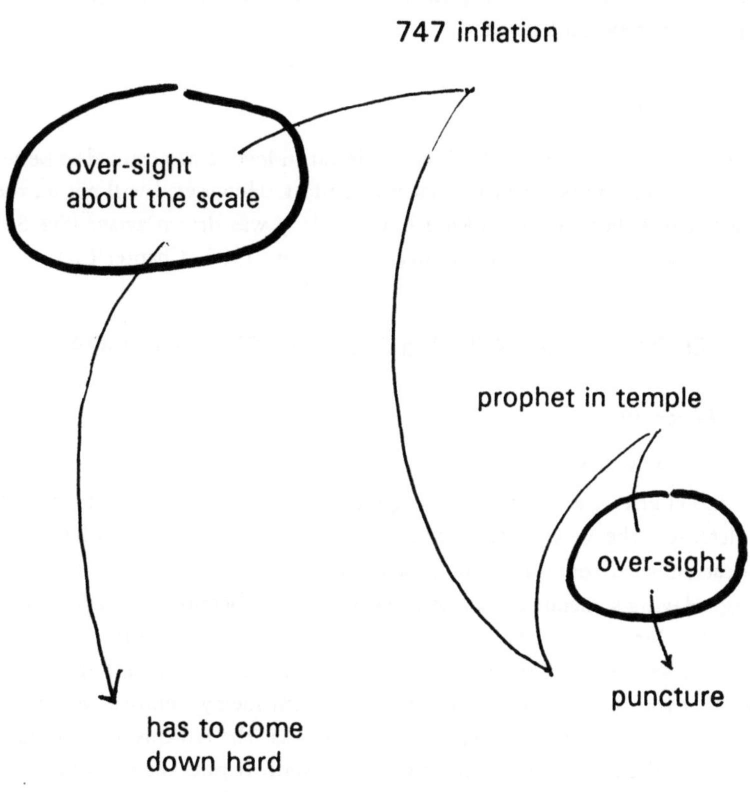

Figure 9.1. The dilemma of the prophet in the temple.

something of his grief and outrage. I would not wait even the length of the first hour to ask him a question, namely, Why had they taken so long to put him in his place? Such a question implies both his considerable talents and his considerable presumption. He confuses heaven and earth. (Myron Sharaf [personal communication] comments that such questions depend upon the *tone.* He finds it safer to get the *history* of the constant attitude [it always will have been adopted in order to survive some evil] in order to call it more gently into question. I felt my patient had so much native strength that I could be sharper with him.)

Other Forms of Presumption

Entitlement comes as well in humbler guises. For example, long-suffering folk may seem to be losers, but can hold forth the catalogue of their woes to outdo Sears. I never wait for more than a half hour. Perhaps I will even raise my hand, like a student in class, to ask if I can ask but one question. Given permission, I may ask but this: "What is your part in this happening over and over again?" This will prove to be a very steadfast curiosity of mine that cannot be dislodged, even when the patient has not the faintest interest in it on his own part. I am not about to be put off from the most important point.

Defeat in Love

A few words on the related subject of defeat in love. I was trained to be terribly sympathetic, and I do believe that that is a comfort. However, I will not let the first hour pass here either without asking how the lady was driven away? (See Sullivan [1956, Chapter 4] for a similar inquiry [Gustafson, 1986, Chapter 6].)

THE SECOND GAP IN THE STORY ON THE SHADOW SLOPE

Reich's Theorem

Reich (1933/1949; Gustafson, 1986, Chapter 4) argued that you do not reach the childhood grief if you cannot challenge the constant attitude, which is the center of all defenses, the very cardinal and substance of the character. Character is an identification with some adult or imagined adult that lifts the child out of his suffering. Having someone to be like gives him a road forward. This adult likeness is likely to win him a place, and the child's abyss will become a thing of the past.

I was never very comfortable with the technical implication of Reich's theorem, namely, that the doctor needed to challenge the attitude by commenting on it in the patient's voice, body posture, and gesture. This was "the red thread" to follow from the surface to the depths of the labyrinth of the soul. It puts the doctor in a godlike position, which weakens the patient's position. Thus, it is easily distorted into a cult of psychotherapy.

I find that my challenge to the patient's amazement on the outer surface, by looking with him at the world, shakes his character, quite like Reich's maneuvers without placing myself over him. We are looking outward together, and I am pointing to a gap in his account. While it is true that this makes me an expert, I am an expert who only proposes, while the patient disposes of what I suggest. He is free to agree or disagree with what I say has been left out.

Once the patient sees his presumption in these overpowering stories (or his subserving in subservience stories, or his delay in delay stories), he is apt to loosen his grip and fall into the shadows from whence he came in his own childhood. The shadow slope in this kind of story can be drastically different from one patient to another. Much can be hidden by a forcing presumption. It is up to us to read it, because the patient will be very frightened and likely to keep us away from his unprotected side as best as he can.

A Case of Jung's Dilemma

My patient, a young teacher, was a kind of prince of doing everything well. This talent got him saddled with every extra responsibility his junior high could put on him. The principal, like Freud, was glad to have a Jung to carry the load of athletics, student government, and science clubs so competently.

He came to me complaining of being absolutely worn out. After he got some

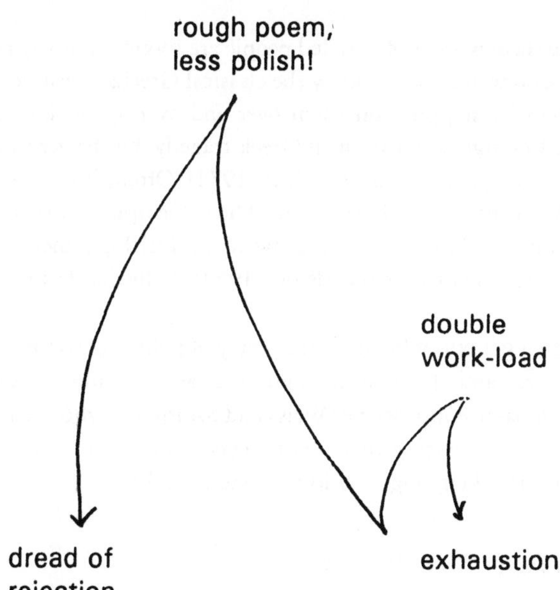

Figure 9.2. Jung's dilemma.

sympathy due from me, I asked him *where* he got the idea that he could handle double the workload of any other teacher in the school? I had put my finger on his presumption, which he didn't much believe in anymore anyway and had begun to feel was pointless. He cried quietly.

I told him I did not think he could live without a god, so we would have to see if another one cropped up in him. Well, it was not long, for he was a writer of poems, and he enjoyed telling me about his craft. Here we came at once to the gap on the shadow slope with the help of a first dream. First dreams are always, to greater or lesser extent, about the fear of this intimate act of sharing dreams (see Chapter 13, "Dream as an Individual Map of Dilemma"). His dream was about showing me a rough poem, whereupon I turned away from him to another patient who had a beautifully finished poem.

His associations were, in brief, that I was a widely educated and polished writer, so I, naturally would prefer a patient like myself. He was very anxious. I replied that he had to be anxious, for he imagined me a kind of Freud that had to have doubles of himself to be appreciative (Newton, 1979). Naturally, this was quite true of his parents, so we had reached his childhood unhappiness.

The gap on the shadow slope for this man is about fear of depending upon someone more powerful than himself because of *their* entitlement! This is not a very difficult transference, for a doctor who is not extremely narcissistic, for he need only show the contrast between this fear and the actual tolerance and even admiration.

Worse Ones

Many of the shadow sides of entitled people are tragic, or nearly tragic, and this is for a simple reason well understood by the classical Greeks. Entitled people pollute those around them by stepping on them over and over again. Sooner or later the offended rise up. Revenge is in the air in Greek tragedy, by the very simple mechanics of pollution-causing resentment (Gardner, 1971). Often, it is the next generation that becomes the agent of the destruction. Thus, Oedipus is cast out to die on a hillside for having a clubfoot, only to grow up to kill his father on the highway without knowing it is his father (Galdston, 1954). Pollution has become suffused, until it explodes.

Children often get out of being at the mercy of polluting parents by identifying with the aggressors, and doing it to their own wives, children, colleagues, and friends. They turn passive into active (Weiss and Sampson, 1986). If I get in the way of this presumption by noticing their drastic effects on everyone around them, they tend to fall back into their tragic childhood vulnerability.

A Case of Polluting or Being Polluted

A middle-aged man came to me in despair because his wife and children were all failing and complaining that it was because of his exacting standards. None of

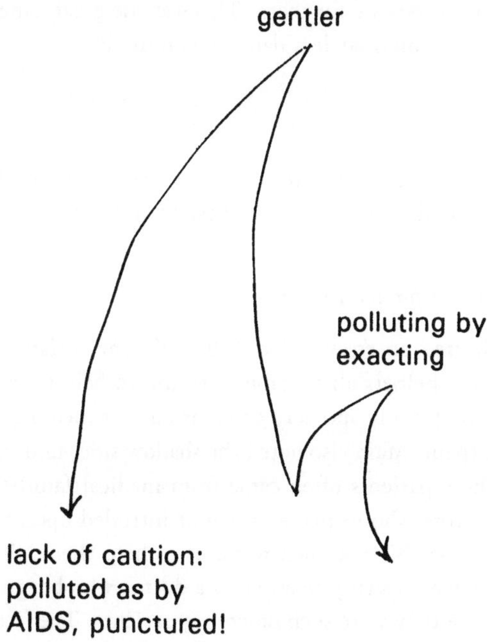

Figure 9.3. A dilemma of polluting or being polluted.

them could live up to his standards, and all were very depressed. The patient was enraged at their backsliding, but was helpless to talk with them. He knew he was polluted with severe disappointment, so anything he said came across as grim and unforgiving. I agreed with him. I was confident that his bitter disappointment went right through walls without his saying a word.

This tragedy, or near tragedy, came from his entitlement to inflict godly demands, as pictured in the famous painting "American Gothic," of the grim couple with the pitchfork, by Grant Wood. An English version is Virginia Woolf's (1927) *To The Lighthouse,* about Mr. Ramsay, a Cambridge professor, and his intimidated children and guests, who cling to Mrs. Ramsay, his mitigating and mild wife.

I felt genuinely sorry for him, yet I also felt he had reaped what he sowed, and I wondered if, as in tragedy itself, his understanding came too late. He backed off his family, but this, naturally, left him with himself as a child. He now recalled what his parents had done to him.

He dreamt he was riding on a train back to his family reunion. The train looked like one from 1950 in Chicago, and he was helping himself through a car by reaching from pole to pole to steady himself. Suddenly, a man put his hand over the patient's own hand on a pole, scratching him. He was terrified, certain he had been given AIDS, and woke up as fast as he could.

The patient was about to go to his family reunion. I told him that his unconscious did not believe he was prepared for these people, who could crush him from the side when he wasn't looking for them. This was the great danger, on the shadow side, now that he was somewhat less dangerous himself.

Seduction

Some of these tragedies are not reparable, yet we are smilingly bidden in. I am getting much better at declining after the first hour at the door.

A Case of Great Honor for the Doctor

I long ago admired an essay called "The Ailment" (Main, 1957), which described patients whose helpers all become ill trying to help them. Main underlines that the patients were queenly and very gracious on first meeting, so that the helper felt lucky to attend them. Main also noted the shadow side, unnoticed because of the sunny welcome. These patients often came from medical families, and were wives and daughters of doctors who neglected them or intruded upon them, so they were polluted with bitterness. No one then was able to help them, their charts grew by the pound, and they were usually referred by a doctor who begged special consideration for them because they were such deserving patients. The fate of foolish helpers was to be punished for their pains, because they could never do enough. The helpers became ill with the ailment, and the patient often committed suicide after finishing off a long line of failing helpers.

In a way, the mechanics of this plot are ridiculously simple, as in the following case. The patient was a middle-aged woman who had been a terrible banshee to her husband and kids but was now reforming, no doubt because they had reached their limits. Her medical doctor called me, and in a charming way told me what a marvelous patient she was in responding to antidepressants. She now had flashbacks to her childhood with her tyrannical father, something like the father in the poetry of Silvia Plath.

I agreed to meet with her to render my opinion. I need not recount the grisly details of her father's mistreatment of her, which were horrible enough. All I need to say is that she smilingly suggested that her medical doctor suggested that I could help her get rid of these inconvenient recollections. What did I think?

In reply, I said that half of the patients with such terrible recollections were relieved by telling somebody about them, and half only felt worse (in Balint's [1968] terms, half are benign and half are malignant). How did she feel having told me about them? To tell the truth, she said, she felt no better at all. I replied that this treatment was not for her, then, unless she felt differently about our talk in the next several weeks. I did not hear from her again, and I was not displeased. Her entire attitude was that she was entitled to miracles and would turn violent when they did not occur on schedule.

The gap on the shadow side, hidden by her charming smile, is her violence,

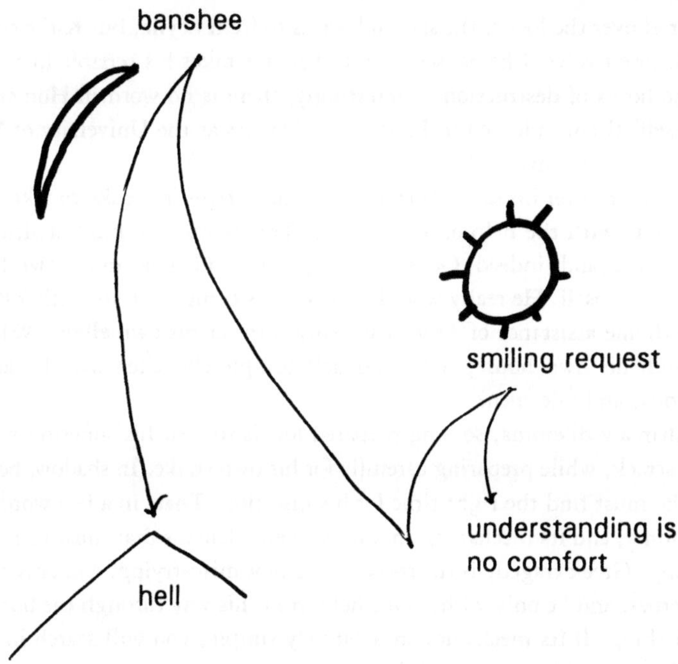

Figure 9.4. A dilemma of great honor for the doctor.

which is turned on me when I cannot perform miracles. I have had five to ten cases of this kind, and now that I read the shadow slope of overpowering stories at the outset, I hope never to have another.

THE THIRD GAP IN THE STORY OF THE PATIENT'S DILEMMA

It would be very nice if it were enough to read the presumption so that it can be let go of, and to read the vulnerability so that it can be felt and grieved and also let go of. It is not this easy, because a dilemma remains that is difficult but often unseen.

This is an ancient dilemma, described over and over in Homer's *Odyssey.* Odysseus, the great hero of the Trojan War, is attempting to get home. He is presumed dead, and suitors devour his household, courting his wife. Penelope is barely holding out, by great wile and courage, and Telemakhos, his son, goes looking for Odysseus.

There are many preparatory dilemmas for Odysseus, such as the great one of Scylla and Kharybdis, where he has to choose between complete destruction in the maelstrom of Kharybdis, or lose six men sweeping by Scylla to her six gullets. He has great grief over the loss of the six, and wants to fight Scylla, but Kirke convinces him he will lose twelve if he pauses to fight her. He takes his terrible loss and sails between the horns of destruction. Interestingly, there is no word in Homer for the situation itself. (I am indebted to Professor of Classics at the University of Wisconsin, Denis Feeney, for his reading of the original Greek.)

In any event, after his series of trials Odysseus arrives in Ithaka to take back his home in secret, with the help of Telemakhos. This is just the kind of situation to drive a hero mad, and, indeed, Odysseus, disguised as a beggar in his own hall, can barely contain himself. He really would have lost his composure altogether if it were not for the divine assistance of Athena at many turns at his own elbow. Who could bear to watch his own house, wife, and hall completely taken over by arrogant, contemptuous, and vile men?

His ultimate dilemma, so long prepared for, is to bear his suffering without a premature attack, while preparing carefully for his own strike. In shadow, he suffers. In reality, he must find the right time for his insertion. That, in a few words, is the classic dilemma, and its mechanics, in a story of entitlement that must ruin itself by overpowering. Greek tragedy is the story of this plot miscarrying, and only the most astute of heroes, and he only with divine help, finds his way through the horns. This is no small thing. If its mechanics are relatively simple, you will search in vain for their full description in the clinical literature.

A Case of a Modern Hero

A very astute female professor came to me very depressed. She had got her family out of a dangerous situation in Latin America, only to be stuck here in a professorship loaded with administrative burdens. She was destroying herself, staying up until two in the morning to write what was important to her, after concluding her duties. She really could not go on like this.

This, in brief, was her dilemma. If she went back to Latin America, where her work was satisfying, her family was endangered. If she stayed here, where her work was onerous, she was endangered. She was already getting sick, and it would get worse with her twenty-hour days.

I noted to her that the obvious escape from the horns of her dilemma was, as for Odysseus, to give up something willingly. What!? If she slighted her administration, the wolves would pounce. I agreed this was not something to risk. Well, she wasn't going to give up her writing, her gardening, her cooking, or excellent mothering. I said that was fine with me, but she was then going to be sick.

She writhed around on my couch. Sliding down the present slope was not sitting well. I said, well, being more modest must be a terrible thing. She laughed, to my relief, and said she'd always, with hard work, done whatever she wanted. And if she could not? Really, it seemed unthinkable to her. I said she must have been a very fortunate (I did not say entitled) being, and she laughed again. I said I did not believe she was capable of being modest, but I was willing to put her to the test.

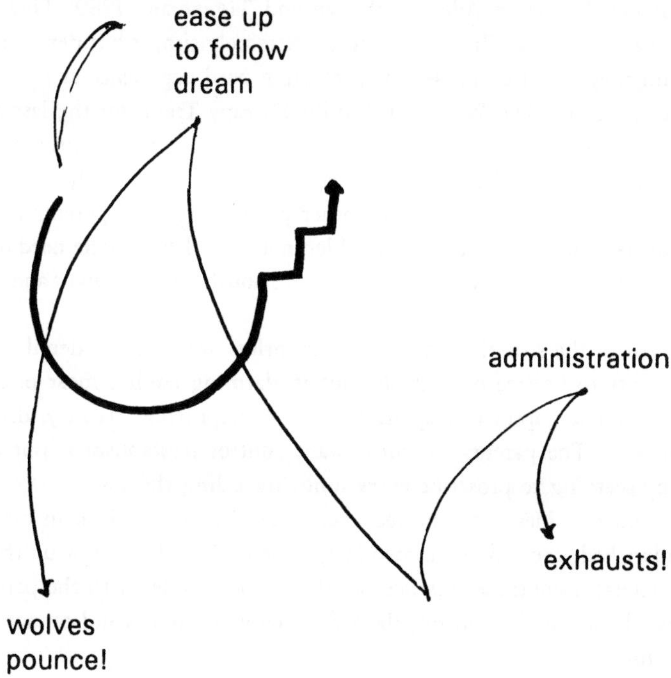

Figure 9.5. A dilemma for a modern Odysseus.

And we would begin by seeing what her unconscious had to say about being a little less ambitious than a queen. Her dreams would tell.

If I had had but a singular idea in a single plan, I would have failed. If caught up in the plane of reality, I had told her this was impossible, she would have felt hurt that I did not appreciate the beauty of her quest as a Renaissance queen, and she would have withdrawn. If caught up in the shadow plane of her injured feelings, I would have been sympathetic to her tears and rage, which would have been comforting, but altered nothing in her entitlement relationship to the world. I hold the two things—her lovely ambition, and her narrow fate with the wolves—together. The first cannot be projected onto the second, and both are crucial, as with Odysseus in his own hall. The mechanics are very simple, but tragic if they are not reckoned as a double description of two absolutely important things, for giving up either is surely ruinous. Her doctor has to see her beautiful and mythical ambition, and her narrow straits. Like Athena for Odysseus, I stand at her elbow.

Parents and Teenagers, and the Dulwich Dilemma

A more banal and completely ordinary dilemma obtains between every vigorous teenager and every parent, and this has been most lucidly appreciated by Australians at the Dulwich Centre in Adelaide (Smith and Tiggeman, 1989; Tiggeman and Smith, 1989) as follows. The mechanics are extremely simple but devastating when missed, and they are often missed. I speak from hard experience as the leader of a family therapy team (The Wisconsin Family Therapy Team) for the last ten years, and from witnessing countless debacles of my students on the horns of the same Dulwich dilemma that they did not (yet) recognize. I routinely deal with this dilemma in individual and brief psychotherapy, talking with parents and talking with teenagers. Since I have gotten the dilemma clear, I have little need of my own team to assist in these cases, which were previously tempestuous and erratic in outcome.

The gist of the situation, despite its countless variations in detail, is that the teenager wants to be free of controls, but is alarming adults, most pointedly his parents, by various lapses of responsibility like shoplifting, truancy, drinking, or what have you. The parents, in turn, want control reestablished, but alarm the teenager by seeming to proscribe everything, including therapy.

If the doctor sides with the teenager's feelings, to join him in his plight of being sandwiched, the parents immediately or soon thereafter throw up their hands, when the teenager continues his license. If the doctor sides with the parents' anxieties to get the kid under control, the kid sullenly withdraws and cannot be moved to do anything.

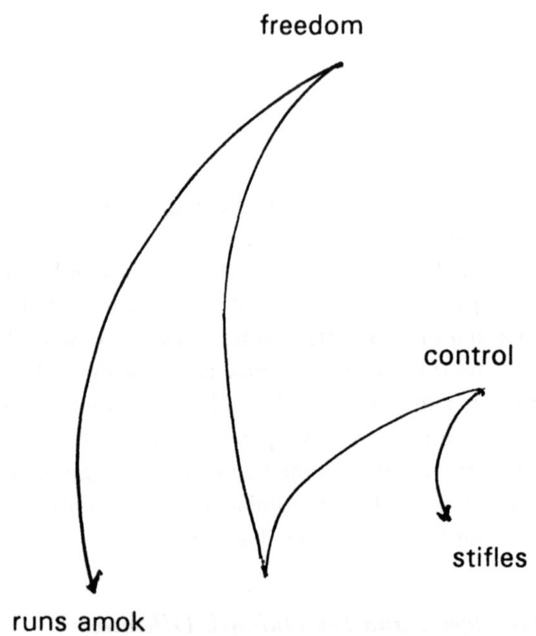

Figure 9.6. The Dulwich dilemma.

Left in this unrepaired confusion the dilemma is terrible, and can run on for the next thirty years, if we leave aside its unmitigated influence on the following generation.

The Dulwich proposal is stunningly simple, catching the opposed principles of freedom for teenagers and control for parents as follows. The doctor says to the teenager after his bitter complaints: Your parents do not believe you can have this freedom so dear to you without misusing it, and going right downhill into a wrecked life. Would you like to prove them wrong? You would? Well, then, what would be evidence persuasive to them that you can use freedom responsibly. What would be a fair test for starters? Essentially, the teenager is obliged to integrate freedom and control to prove the parents wrong.

Similarly, the doctor turns to the parents as follows: Your teenager believes that you cannot relinquish control at all, which will ruin his life. Would you like to prove him wrong? You would? What then would be evidence persuasive to him that you can give up some control? What would be a fair test for starters? Essentially, the parent is obliged to integrate control and freedom to prove the teenager wrong.

It usually takes a number of sessions beyond the proposal of the first for the various tests, slips, excesses, yelling, and anxieties to occur. I find that the Dulwich proposal of the dilemma makes the dilemma solvable in three of four controversies of the kind. (Of course, it is important to understand the one out of four that remains intransigent. See Selvini-Palazzoli *et al.* [1989] and the next section of this chapter.)

It is very important to add something, which takes another three or four or five years to make evident. The teenager continues in his dilemma. This is because freedom is a mythical delight, and control is a cruel necessity that has a place in the world. Some teenagers gravitate toward subserving, some delaying their beautiful ideal, and some insist on forcing it on others in their entitlement. It is the very difficult task of growing up to find a balance between demands and responsibilities, and getting through the big fight with the parents in high school is but one chapter in a long story.

Paradox, or Selvini's Dilemmas

In conclusion, I need to say something about marriage, a complex subject in which I must be competent to do individual brief psychotherapy, since it, like children, is one of the main subjects of complaint and conversation. Entitlement is its chief controversy. My entitlement is apt to be at my wife's expense, and hers at mine, since somebody has to take care of business while somebody is fulfilling themselves. More deeply, everyone is entitled to a better spouse. That is because we are all mismatched. We have mistaken our spouses for our perfect double, and in every case we find that they meet only some of our needs.

This gives rise to what Selvini-Palazzoli *et al.* (1978) call the paradox of very difficult marriages (I think it is there in all marriages), which she and her colleagues

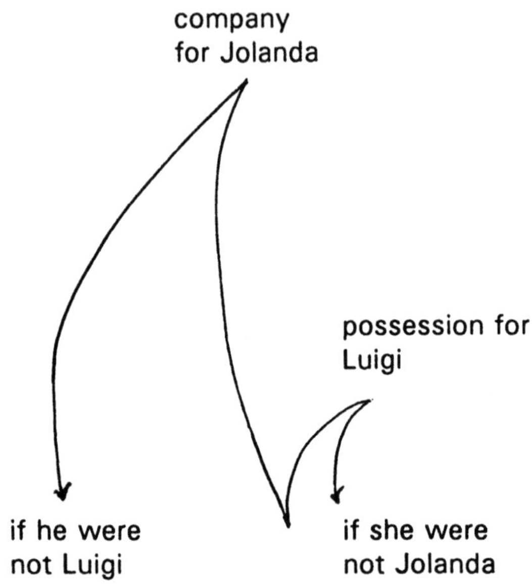

Figure 9.7. Selvini's dilemma.

were at one time wont to spell out for the couple by announcing it as something required. One of my favorite paradoxes is this pair of letters to be read aloud:

> Luigi,
>
> I do not see you, I don't hear you, because I'm not even here. I'm with Doctor Selvini. I'm doing this for you, because if I were to show you how much I love you, I would put you in an intolerable position.
>
> Jolanda,
>
> I can't say that I have hostile feelings for Doctor Selvini because, even if I did, and if I said so, it would be the same as saying I love you, and this would put you in an intolerable position. (Selvini-Palazzoli et al., 1978, p. 133).

My point is not a technical one about whether to announce such things or not (Selvini has gone on to other maneuvers; a paradox, in any event, is a denied dilemma), but rather I am pointing to the structural dilemma in the marriage. Jolanda is in a very routine dilemma of women needing more company than their husbands, even being entitled to more company than their husbands, but feeling pinned down by them. Luigi is in a very routine dilemma of resenting his wife's extra needs out of his entitlement to have her to himself, but in no way being prepared to meet her needs himself!

Technically speaking, I am inclined simply to present the dilemma without the legerdemain.

The Case of a Drinking Husband, or the Irish Dilemma

Very simply, the wife had an alcoholic and violent father, so any whiff of this substance from her husband gave her great distress, and she felt entitled to have a marriage without alcohol. I certainly sympathized with her. In turn, her husband, being a decent and hard-working man, felt entitled, if somewhat guiltily, to a beer or two after work to release him from the great strain of his day in the factory. I certainly sympathized with him.

Of course, to side with one or the other would be disastrous. I simply told the more entitled of the two, the wife, that the drinking certainly was not all right with her, period, but that giving up this dear man was not going to be all right either. What did she propose to do? She cried, and rightly so, because there was going to be great pain for her either way. That is a typical problem of entitlement in a marriage. I construe it in terms of the dilemma that is implicit but often overlooked, just because it is too hard to face up to without help.

Chapter 10

More Complex Idealists

Idealists stand apart from the world in the name of their ideal, but this is not, in itself, complex. The ideal is likely to be a simple elaboration that is served by the patient. In other words, idealism is usually a story of subservience, with its usual dilemma and fate, as described in Chapter 7.

There is a difference between a sketchy ideal and one that is dwelt upon at great length and thus elaborated. As Edelman (1979, 1982, 1985, 1989) argues in his group selection theory of the brain, the more a subject is utilized, the more its group of cells in the brain literally expands. And further, the larger the area of the brain devoted to the ideal, the less quickly it will go away. In biological terms, it becomes more robust (Allen and Starr, 1982).

In other words, idealists resist change. It is important for the practice of psychotherapy to distinguish the motives for idealism. I will distinguish three motives for standing apart in a relatively simple way, and elaborating a very lengthy idealism, which is just the same idea over and over again in slightly different variations. With these types in mind, we can go on to see what actual complex idealism looks like, and what its challenges are in both long and brief psychotherapy. Perhaps, I should say that actual complexity involves at least two ideas that do not fit together very well. The individual has to wrestle with them.

THREE MOTIVES FOR LENGTHY IDEALISM

The three great motives for idealism are admiration, pain, and entitlement. When only one of the three motives drives the idealism, it repeats itself and is thus entirely redundant.

Admiration

Some children come from families with beliefs that are beautiful to them, and they hold onto them despite collisions with the world. They have been blessed with enough support, like some of those black children who withstood the violent racist crowds in the first days of school integration in the South.

The great force that inspires these children is a kind of god, although not all of them would use religious terms to characterize their faith. They have values that they will not surrender to getting on in the world. These values lead to creation of a world elsewhere (Poirier, 1966).

A relatively straightforward example is the great Scottish Olympic runner Eric Liddell, as shown in the movie *Chariots of Fire,* who shows enormous courage to go his own way. He refuses to run on Sunday, yielding his chance at perpetual worldly glory. He also opposes his family, who want him to give up his training for missionary work in China. He replies to his sister:

> But I've got a lot of running to do first. Jennie, you've got to understand. I believe that God made me for a purpose . . . for China. He also made me fast. And when I run I feel His pleasure. To give it up would be to hold him in contempt. To win is to honor Him.

An individual like this has to stay with his God, however different it makes him, for it shines through him. If he gives it up, it is like turning out the light forever. Fortunately, a runner named Lindsay gives up his place to Liddell in a different race that is not on Sunday. Two members of the Olympic Committee, Effie and George, discuss the close call as follows:

EFFIE: A sticky moment, George . . . Thank God for Lindsay. I thought the laddie had us beaten.

GEORGE: He did have us beaten, Effie, and thank God he did!

EFFIE: I don't think I quite follow you.

GEORGE: The laddie, as you call him, is a true man of spirit and a true athlete. His speed is a mere extension of his life, its force. We sought to sever his running from his self.

EFFIE: For his country's sake, yes.

GEORGE: No sake is worth that, Effie, least of all a guilty national pride.

This George is a gem, for he understands spirit, while Effie is the commonplace, worldly man who has not got a clue of what it's all about.

We never talk about spirit in psychiatry. It is even strange to place spirit and psychiatry in the same sentence. We feel their repulsion of each other. The dictionary definition of spirit is lengthy, running on to thirty-one meanings, suggesting it is a very meaningful idea. The first definition is "the principle of conscious life; the vital principle in man, animating the body or mediating between body and soul." The idea is an ancient one, coming from the Latin word *spirare,* to breathe or to blow. This is the very sense in which George uses the term. The Holy Spirit is what makes the man go.

Of course, psychiatry cannot discuss the condition of the spirit because it is wholly given to looking at man from the *outside* as an *object*. To help people like Eric Liddell, you need to enter into his nature as a subject, as a spirit inspired by a Spirit.

Jung (1925/1971) is one of the few psychiatrists who did understand spirit and its relation to Spirit, so he is practically the only guide with a map of idealism and its aberrations. Essentially, Jung argues that there are many gods besides the well-known Holy Spirit of Eric Liddell. Jung wrote that often the individual cannot tell you what the god is that inspires him. Often, the individual is possessed by the god to do its bidding, to the detriment of the individual.

A Case of Atlas

This doctor came to me in a rage, because her clinic was throwing her out as a troublemaker. She could not believe that they would do this to her. After all, she had the highest standards of medicine and did twice the amount of work of anybody there. She was amazed that such virtue would be tossed out. She was the very underpinning of the Clinic, that which held it up. Like the idealist Lydgate, in George Eliot's *Middlemarch,* she was of the highest temper, and hardly anybody could stand her.

To make twenty sessions very brief, I tackled her amazement at the Clinic

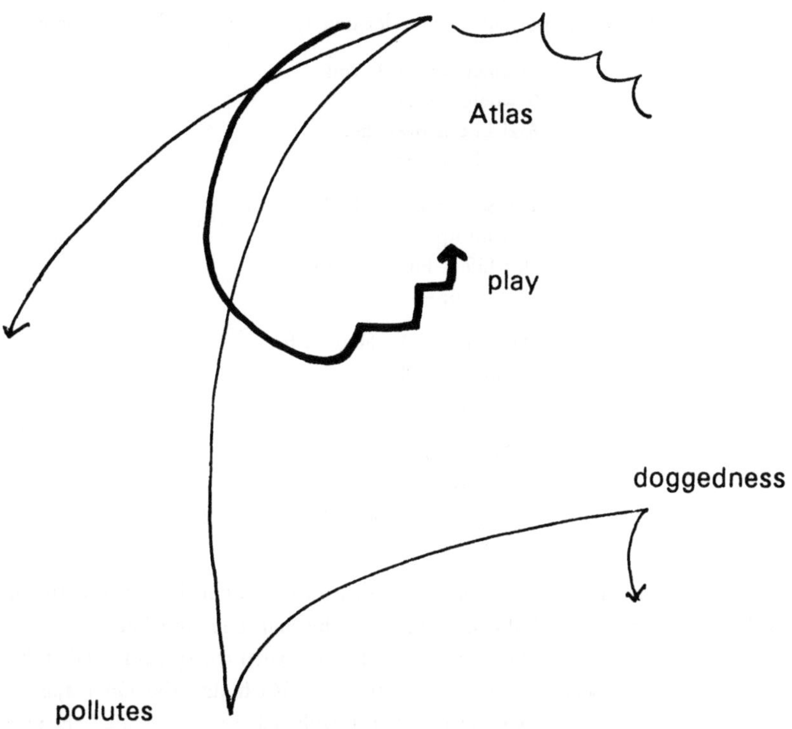

Figure 10.1. Can Atlas play?

wanting to be rid of her. There was nothing amazing about it all, for she was on everybody's case, and they could hardly like her for dogging them. Luckily, she had a sense of humor, so I could get her to laugh when I caught her berating people over and over, which she could hardly help doing. I would say something like, "Oh, that's surprising," and she would smile. There was a little play in this system, which I could extend.

This was only half the work. I had to start at the outer surface of her collisions with the world, but I had to get to the inner surface of the inspiration that drove her outward. As Jung (1916/1972) wrote, it is easiest to demonstrate this from dreams, where the god will appear in person. Not all patients can give me dreams, and she could not. We got to her god, from her reading about a particular physician who, if not a god, was a demigod, an Atlas. She had to be like him, beautiful as he was to her in his huge energy. I could wholly admire this inspiration, while having doubts, aloud, about running headlong in it at the world. She gradually got her balance. After all, she could do what he did but more quietly, without inflicting it on one and all.

Pain

The second motive is the pain or even dread of being near other people, having been so injured by them, perhaps most eloquently put by Emily Dickinson:

> I cannot live with You
> It would be Life—
> And Life is over there
> Behind the Shelf
>
> The Sexton keeps the Key to—
> Putting up
> Our Life—His Porcelain—
> Like a Cup—
>
> Discarded of the Housewife—
> Quaint or Broke
>
> * * *
>
> So We must meet apart—
> You there—I here
> With just the Door ajar
> That Oceans are . . .

I have left out some difficult lines in the middle of the poem about the vulnerability of the lady to intrusion and abandonment by the man courting her.

When this vulnerability is true with everyone, then the subject needs take up a half-in and half-out position with everyone . . . "With just the Door ajar / That Oceans are . . . ," and this is what Guntrip (1968, Chapter 30) called the schizoid position. Some people in the schizoid position have a sketchy inner world, some elaborate one idea, and some develop many ideas, as Dickinson did. Thus, the position is sterile repetition if it contains no other idea than taking the position itself, while it can be fertile when also inspired, like Dickinson, by the transcendent glory of creation. All become their own company, or find company in nature or in their libraries.

A Case of Escher, Repeated

This woman was a younger sister, like Cinderella, left out of the alliance of the big sisters and the mother. She learned to subserve to have a place at all. She had a secret world of art, in which she was well versed. It never got out of her sketchbooks, because she felt so big and powerful doing it that it made her dizzy. She would do a little, and then set it aside.

Thus, she was either other-absorbed and vacant and weary, or self-absorbed and full and frighteningly energetic, with almost nothing in between. She loved Escher, because it was about the only mapping she ever saw of the stairways and tunnels and reversals between the perspective of others and the perspective of oneself that are incompatible.

My work with her could not be brief, because of this dilemma. Both horns were untenable—the perspective of others, and her perspective of herself. She could, slowly, as she trusted me to understand the situation, show me how she got from one

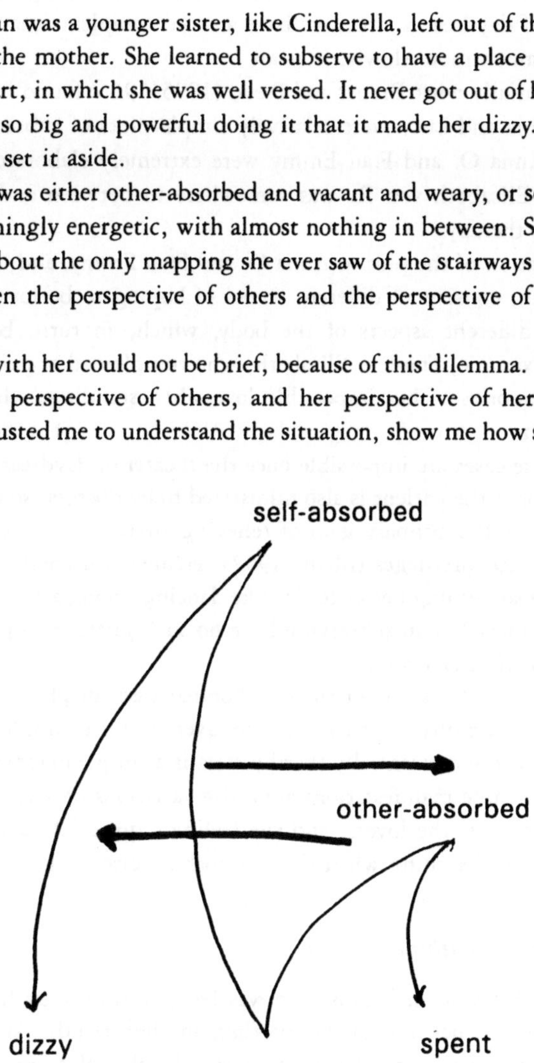

Figure 10.2. Escher's opposing currents.

untenable slope to the other, like Escher himself. Her dichotomous world was shared and so slightly less painful. It was a little like the Cheshire Cat showing up for Alice, that is, to comfort and orient her, and that is a big thing.

Entitlement

Everyone who is ill-used in their service to others will develop a compensatory dream that is also dangerous in its claims. As I described in Chapter 7, this is the simple dilemma of subservience. If the compensatory dream is highly elaborated in a kind of theater of daydreams, then we have a more complex situation, which will yield its claims much more slowly, if at all.

This is essentially what Breuer and Freud (1895/1966) found in their *Studies on Hysteria*. Katharina and Lucy were relatively simple plots of subservience for brief therapy, while Anna O. and Frau Emmy were extremely elaborated and went on endlessly, while Elisabeth von R. was somewhere in between and ended up as a successful longer therapy.

This elaboration of the plot in Anna O. and Frau Emmy, and to a lesser extent Fraulein Elisabeth, consists of different scenes of hoping to be loved, that become associated with different aspects of the body, which, in turn, become different symptoms. For example, Fraulein Elisabeth, who complained of pains in the thigh, had different memories of her impossible love when standing, when sitting, and when lying down.

Most of these cases are impossible once the theater of daydreams has become a way of life, and once the patient is also ministered to by doctors, so that the case has what the analysts call a primary gain of relieving anxiety and a secondary gain of being rewarded with privileges (Main, 1957). Fraulein Elisabeth came out of her dilemma, having something better to do, like dancing, being attractive, and rejoining society, but many lost in subserving have no such glittering opportunity. They acquire a medical theater instead.

Therefore, when I see one of these elaborated cases of physical complaints, I contemplate most carefully whether there are avenues for a simpler but gratifying life. Sullivan (1956) said essentially that hysteria is a simple diagram made complicated by fantasy, whose manifestations are really variations on a theme, with minor changes in the setting, the lovers, and the feelings, quite like a soap opera. This activity is endlessly absorbing when there is nothing else to do.

A Case of a Duchess without a Duchy

I first saw this woman because she was being run over by her husband, her daughters, her bosses, her mother, her brother, and her friends. All took advantage of her good nature. So far we have just a simple plot of subservience. But she developed an array of physical complaints, an appetite for staying in bed and reading

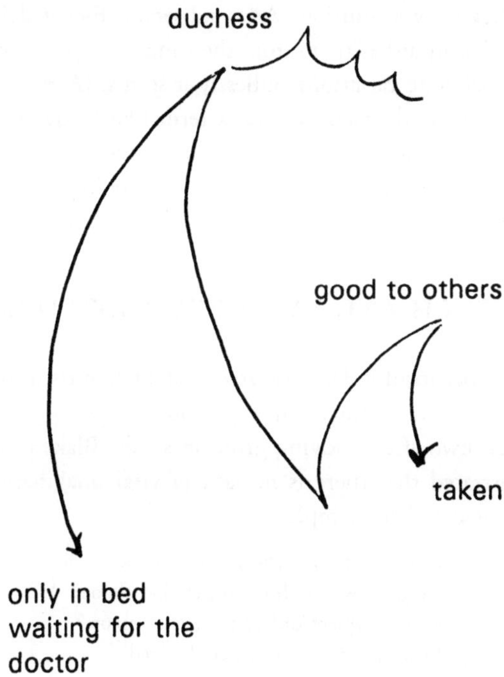

Figure 10.3. A duchess in bed.

love stories, and a capacity for bumbling in her work as a saleswoman. Naturally, she became a fascinating medical case, for it was her best chance to shine, and she did.

Male Versions

I would not like to leave the impression that women are the only culprits in this kind of plot. Our Veterans Hospital is a veritable temple for disadvantaged men who, perhaps more quietly than women, develop their medical careers, often for lack of a better opportunity. The histories are redundant. They have been struck down sticking up for themselves, often very sincerely, even patriotically, in the armed services. Coming back to peacetime with high hopes, they are dashed again, at work and with their wives, and even their children and their friends. Then the elaborate medical career begins.

Copying

Atlas, Escher, and the Duchess all have a grand vision but must live in a little world. There is a psychic inflation (Jung, 1971) in the vision, and a psychic deflation in the actual. What do they do with this dilemma?

Essentially, they copy a solution. Atlas subserves; Escher delays; the Duchess overpowers. What distinguishes them from the simplest types is the energy of their composition; they elaborate variations endlessly it seems. (A *melisma* is the simplest copying device in the parody mass, taking a term like Kyrie and repeating it for fifteen minutes! [Ruth Gustafson, personal communication]. The urge to copy can be extremely strong, in music as in life.) The results are highly stable, and thus are little altered by us.

THE FRENCH AND SAINT-EXUPERY'S DILEMMA

Gilligan (1990) has beautifully demonstrated that little girls of ten are naturalists full of curiosity and delight in their own expression. By having both boys and girls write poems of their own after studying great ones, like Blake's "The Tyger," Koch (1973) has demonstrated that there is no lack of vital imagination in children of elementary school grades. For example:

Dog, where did you get that bark?
Dragon, where did you get that flame?
Kitten, where did you get that meow?
Rose, where did you get that red?
Bird, where did you get those wings?
DESIREE LYNNE COLLIER

You can keep this imagination going in children simply by giving them a place to keep talking and writing about what they see. Gilligan did this in Boston by having the girls talk about such things as the women painted by male artists in the Boston Museum of Fine Arts; Koch did it in his poetry classes; the Young Shakespeare Players do it here in Madison, performing plays and discussing them as they go.

The trouble is that such liberal education has to collide with the world sooner and later. By following her girls, Gilligan found that they began to say "I don't know" with exponential frequency between the ages of ten and fifteen, to fit into the girl packs that did not like girls who talked in an individual way. They were practicing becoming objects for men. In *Le Petit Prince,* St. Exupery tells a parallel tale of a boy with an imagination trying to fit into a world of men who care only for their numbers in their increase packs.

I call it the French dilemma, not because it is confined to France, but because it has been so clearly understood by a series of French writers from Montaigne and Pascal to Rostand and St. Exupery. The dilemma is this. You can retire from the world into your beautiful study to read and ponder or write, as Pascal (1662/1966) wrote: "I have often said that the sole cause of man's unhappiness is that he does not know how to stay quietly in his room." He is echoing the sentiments of Marcus Aurelius, a most respected Roman Emperor, who wrote: "This is the secret of cheerfulness, of depending on no help from without and needing to crave from no man the boon of tranquility." (The source of these two quotations and their linkage is Michael Moran [personal communication].) However you still have to come down from this study into the world. The French essayist Montaigne had a library with a gallery in a tower, in which he could pace while he thought, but he had to come down and face the brigands who were rampaging in his neighborhood.

When you come down to the world, you encounter raw energy flowing forcefully in channels, which I have described as increase packs: Montaigne's brigands taking whatever they can lay their hands on, and nowadays slightly more civilized packs, increasing their numbers of contracts, patients, students, papers, investigations, and so forth. The social world flows crudely by formula, as it always has.

The dilemma of the child-adult who is a naturalist, who likes her own curiosity, and who does not want to surrender herself to the prevailing formula concerns the compromise that will be made with it. Turquet (1975), another French (and English, by immigration) writer, argued that there were only three possible compromises. The first is to submit altogether and become a member who surrenders individual expression almost entirely—what he called a membership-individual. The second is to refuse to submit at all and remain idiosyncratic and apart—what he called a singleton. The third is to insist on individual expression in some ways, while submitting to the requirements of membership in other ways—what he called an individual-member. Of course, there are shadings of gray along this continuum, from absolute singularity to the midpoint of individual-membership to the absolute disappearance of self in membership.

Of course, being fond of self-expression keeps you apart, like Rostand's *Cyrano,* who throws over the comedy because it is not to his taste. He is an extravagant army of one, overturning an entire culture that is sinking into base and material acquisition in favor of his devotion to the perfect Lady. He is a medieval knight, fighting a hopeless battle against the modern tide that flows into formulae for increasing territory.

St. Exupery's Little Prince is a similar knight, in terms of values. He too wishes to love, and be loved, more than anything. He loves his rose, and later his fox, and they him. He too encounters *les grandes personnes,* who care only for their formulae of increasing, like the astronomer his planets, the king his subjects, the tipler his admirers, and so forth. Like Cyrano, the Little Prince hasn't a chance in the world of overturning these theaters. Each theater is an asteroid in firm control of one of the specialists. The Little Prince ends up leaving this world for his star, apart and dying.

St. Exupery's variation of the French dilemma is that there is a terrible fall from childhood grace to adult numbers, and that the latter formula will budge for no man or woman. If you have the numbers, you are in, and if you don't you are out. Cyrano is in, only if enough people go to the theater to watch him. The Little Prince is in, on the same basis. A complex personality, or individual-member, has to reach across that chasm, surrendering neither himself nor his grasp of the numbers.

A Case of a Viking Prince

This man was a somewhat original photographer, who showed up late to work repeatedly and got fired. He had a childhood in which his father had no interest for his pursuits but only wanted him to toe the line, which he didn't, and thus he got put down repeatedly.

He had a very beautiful dream, in which he was looking out from a second-story window at a parade in a big city, the miracle being that a Viking ship was sailing right down the avenue before his eyes. The avenue was called Jackson Street. His association to Jackson Street was Jack Johnson, the Norwegian boxer, his childhood hero to replace his father.

His dilemma was that he had to hold onto this glory, like Cyrano or the Little Prince, or his light would go out, and he had to get to work on time or his father and his father-successors, like the bosses, would quash him.

My job was to pose the problem, the *reach* he needed between his vision and his actual place. He responded by putting together a beautiful show that met the guidelines for exhibition in a certain gallery. He had a beautiful dream, in which he was a carpenter putting up a stage. He did not occupy the Shakespearean stage himself, this belonging to others, but only a little place in the back, which was intricate and beautiful to him, like something out of Samuel Beckett.

The unanticipated setback was that the gallery folded for its own financial reasons before the show, leaving him heartbroken and in the lurch. He then dreamt of falling downstairs in a Roman villa in an orgy of license, exaggerating his distress into an agony of suicide. Obviously, he was playing an old role to the hilt, that of making things worse than they were, hoping to get his mother's sympathy.

Of course, I was dealing with a pair of transferences. Rejected by his father, he invented a new father-god, Jack Johnson (A). This crashed against the mundane requirements. With my help, he made a compromise of bringing himself down to scale, a Beckett in the corner (C). When this was dashed, he made himself much worse, just as he had as a child appealed to his mother to rescue him from fatherly requirements (B). I was not impressed that he was so bad, nor was I going to fall into being that mother. I shared his pain with him, admitted his bad luck, and pointed back the way into another contest.

The patient's comments upon my original draft discussing his dilemma clarify his fragility, which I understated:

> I was in awe of the ship and wanted just a little piece of it, but as I stepped closer to examine the planking it seemed flawed—nonetheless still huge and unobtainable . . .
>
> And you have helped me to see the need to play Becket . . . but I'm not sure I have made it my show yet. . . .
>
> When I let go of all that, this empty feeling—and fear of going mad tends to replace it. Now I am just trying to hang on . . .
>
> (signed) THE LITTLE PRINCE

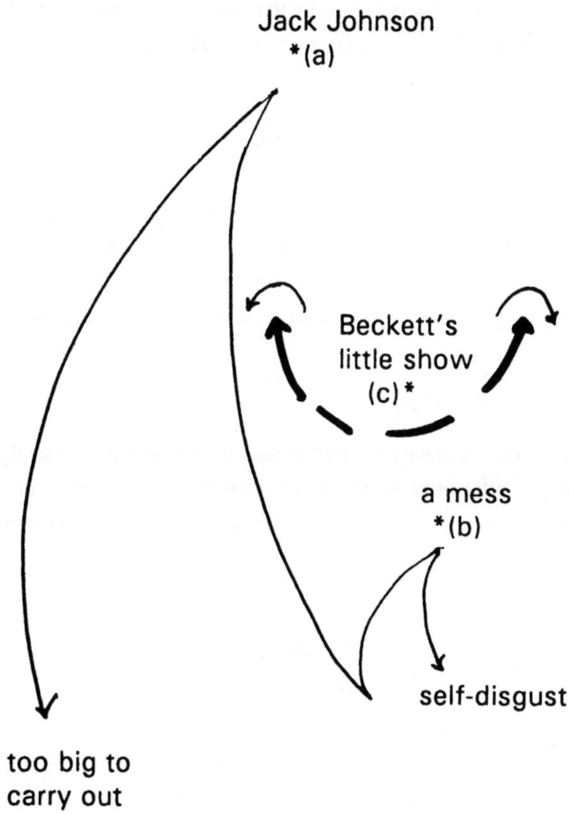

Figure 10.4. How big a prince?

In summary, he cannot be Jack Johnson (A), and he cannot be completely pathetic (B), and he imagines a middle-sized stage for himself (C), but that too is unstable. Typically, these cases take a very long time to stabilize. I have a great many of them, which constitute my practice of long-term psychotherapy. Essentially, I am most helpful when I am extremely clear that A and B will never work, and that C is possible but may drift back into A of grandiosity or B of inadequacy. Gradually C emerges as a third thing, with its own practices and accomplishness and relationships.

In terms of catastrophe theory (Callahan and Sashin, 1990), there are two cusps that are pulling for the patient, grandiosity and inadequacy. The region in between hardly exists. The ability to contain feelings by discussing them, dreaming them, and picturing them creates the third region. Of course, C emerges to varying degrees, depending upon the strength of the patient's constitution or vitality, the "play" in his system as opposed to rigidity, the availability of company in which to display this play, and the availability of work in which to triumph. However, this discussion of long-term work is beyond the scope of this book, and I will take it up in my next book *Brief Versus Long Psychotherapy* (1995).

TIMING

I have seen the Viking Prince once a month for two years, or twenty-four sessions, and I expect we will continue for several more years. For him, that is the necessary pace needed to crystallize a third structure (C) to transcend his dilemma (A and B). Others are ready to go once a week, and to arrive rapidly at C and to conclude.

The Case of the Gigantic Carrot

I saw this woman once every two weeks for twelve sessions. Again, she chose the pace. Usually, I offer once a month, or once every two weeks, or once a week, to indicate a range. I am willing to extend the range, however, to once every several

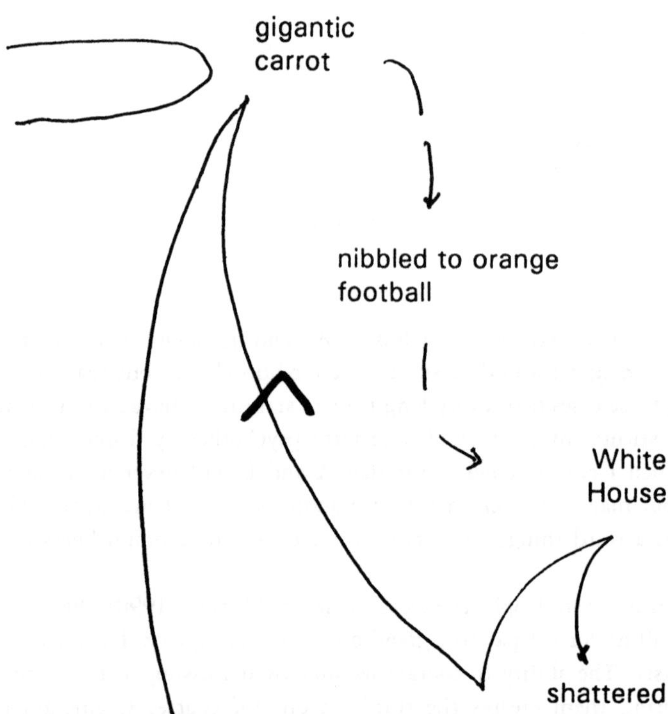

Figure 10.5. The fertility of the gigantic carrot.

months, thinning it out, or twice a week, thickening the intensity. I am quite convinced, like Winnicott was (Gustafson, 1986, Chapter 7), that the tempo of individuation is best decided by the patient.

I will be a little schematic about our very imaginative series of discussions, to show the transition that she made from early to middle to late sessions.

An early dream was of her being in her childhood home, but it was surrounded and circled by broken glass and a gang of dangerous men she had to go out and negotiate with. This, ever so briefly, took us to the shattering of the beautiful stained glass of her childhood dream to be perfectly married; her marriage was now in ruins and she in grief.

A middle dream was of a gigantic carrot growing out from her house and under the sidewalk, where it was being excavated. It had been nibbled by some animal to the size of an orange football. This, ever so briefly, took us to her rage at letting her fertility be chewed without a return to her.

In a late dream, she was climbing up into a beautiful fire tower, with a new man in her life reaching down to pull her in, only he was "ham-handed." That is, his hands were big and clumsy and crude, and she was very uncomfortable and anxious. This, ever so briefly, took us to her longing to find her double, which, her unconscious told her, this man was not.

There is a lot I could say about all this, but I do not want to be diverted from the formula of complexity I am trying to keep before the reader. It is the French or St. Exupery's dilemma. Creation, such as her carrot, is one beautiful thing, and crossing the chasm to reach the world across the sidewalk is another, where glass is smashed, animals nibble you down to a football, and ham-hands pull you into bed.

Strength

This patient had been deeply loved as a child, so that she left me readily, once we had helped her create these maps of crossing from her beauty into the world. She just went ahead, forewarned and forearmed. Of course, many patients did not have this security as a child. If they find an ally in me, which they have hardly had before, they can build a similar and beautiful map, but they cannot forswear my company in St. Exupery's dilemma. It is too terrifying on their own.

A Case of the Black Madonna

This young woman had married into a very hard-nosed family that she was no match for, quite like the Wilcoxes, the auto-manufacturers who always got their way in E. M. Forster's *Howard's End.* Trampled too many times, bruised, ignored, and unheeded, she moved to Madison to get away from them, separating on a kind of trial basis from her husband.

The story of her psychotherapy is long, at twice a week early on and once a week later for four years, which is what I want to explain, as simply as I can. A dream, I

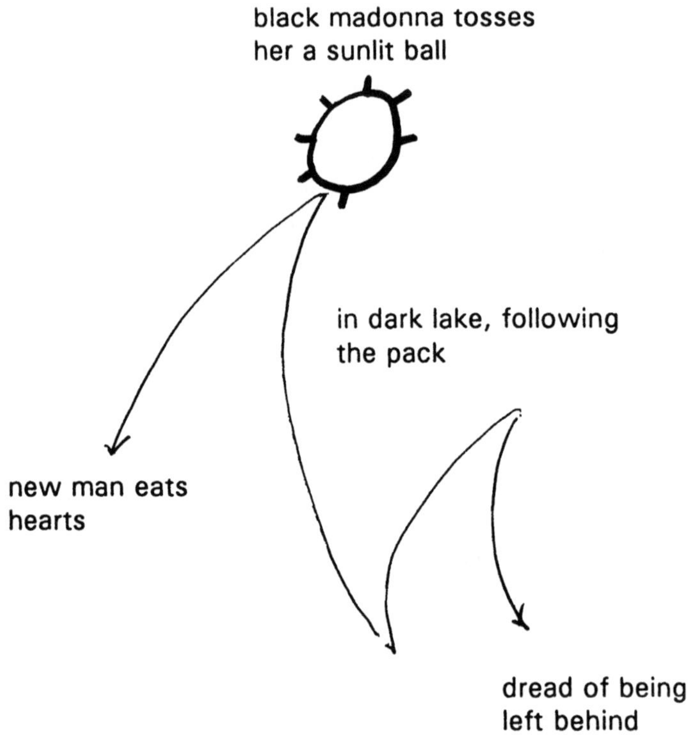

Figure 10.6. Company from the black madonna.

hope will make the point. She was following a band of Indians walking in a lake up to their chests, in darkness and silence, toward a Capitol on a distant horizon. She dreaded getting too far behind them, as she might step into a hole and drown. Of course, this was a vivid picture of surviving, barely, in the increase pack of her in-laws, fearing to separate from them altogether and go under.

Then, she somehow found herself floating on her back in the water, pointed backwards, quite at ease. Through her toes, she sighted a beautiful black girl with a beach ball standing in the lake. The girl said, "Where are you going, lady?" with a smile, and popped the beach ball up into the air, where the sun's rays caught it with astonishing beauty.

She was very moved by her own creation of the dream, which reminded me of the black madonna in Chartres, a figure of great encouragement to women at sea in a dark and dangerous world of war. Again, I want to stay with my formula of complexity, the dilemma of St. Exupery, about the chasm between sunlit creation like this, and living with the silent, trodding pack in the dark lake.

This is the long-term version of St. Exupery's dilemma. The creation is beautiful, but the ability to protect herself from the crudeness of men is slow to occur.

Chapter 11

More Complex Detours

Everyone has had the painful experience of having something precious, and showing it to someone else who finds it worthless. This is why interest is dangerous, for it can confirm what is loved as beautiful, or it can disconfirm it as undeserving. Thus, we all learn to delay showing our favorite possessions.

Some of us have been so wounded that we never show our actual concerns at all, but play a false self (Winnicott, 1971a) perpetually. The true self is apart, in the clouds or in some other unreachable place. This can appear to be complicated. Actually, it is not. The self apart elaborates one idea over and over, of grandiosity in the form of the self as one god or another, which is what Jones (1923) called the God complex.

When there is only one idea, the idea is presented as plus, minus, and somewhere in between. For example, I can fantasize I am a triumphant Super Man, a Super Man about to be killed by Evil Incarnate, or some mixture of the two, with the outcome still in doubt. Of course, sometimes, the saga is hidden, as in the disguise of the mundane Clark Kent, mild-mannered reporter who seems to be a nobody. This is the formula of the modern detective story since A. C. Doyle's Sherlock Holmes. While the details can approach infinity, the elaboration hardly alters the single idea of the plot.

Since everyone seems to get a thrill out of these stories, it is to be inferred that everyone has some interest in himself or herself as a hidden god. Everyone has some delay, of a secret grandiosity. The fully false self is altogether split between a false show of being what is required in society and a true self wholly given over to grandiose pretensions (compare the schizoid position, which is half mask and half disclosure).

Before we get to the actual complexity of delay, which requires at least two ideas, let us visit the pseudo-complexity of a God complex as one idea reiterated.

THREE KINDS OF ELABORATE DELAY

Grandiosity

The Case of Freud's Wolf Man (1918)

This was a kind of detective story like the combination of Sherlock and Sigmund in the modern movie *The Seven Per Cent Solution,* only this extremely elaborate

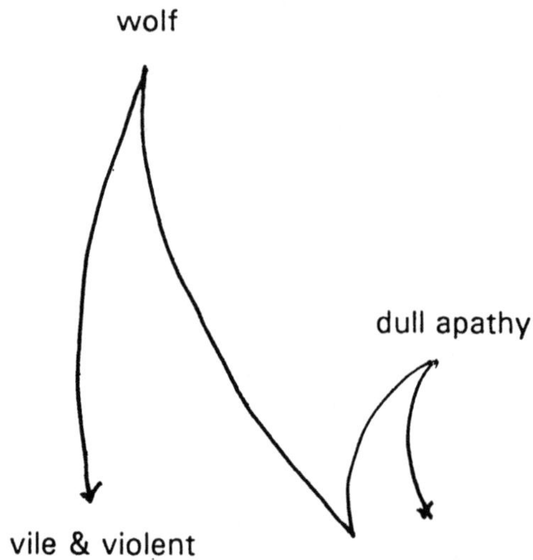

Figure 11.1. The dilemma of the Wolf Man.

clinical variation has the hero, Freud, underestimate his quarry, the Wolf Man. This quarry, actually a patient, was a very disturbed man—grandiose, manic-depressive, paranoid—who gave Freud a beautiful dream of wolves, thus earning him his name. Freud hoped to fully analyze the dream and release the patient from his labyrinthine neurosis. Freud did succeed in a brilliant analysis of the dream, and in setting an end to the treatment, but the patient remained as grandiose and insane as ever. Freud ended up taking collections to support his famous patient, who could not work but felt entitled to the doctor looking after him (Gardner, M., 1971)!

Freud's marvelous sleuthing of the dream I have tracked elsewhere (Gustafson, unpublished a), and I will not repeat it because it is not to our purpose. Suffice it to say that it is a nightmare of the boy looking out his bedroom at a tree full of white wolves staring at him in complete silence. The dream has enormous allusions, all of which are tracked beautifully to their sources. The point is that this boy-man has one idea that proves indestructible, of his being entitled to complete attention. When the attention is taken from him, he becomes vile and violent. When this mood passes, he is in dull apathy, and can hardly move himself to do anything, even to lift a finger to take care of himself.

This is not a plot that any doctor is going to free any patient from, not even the great Freud. The man's dilemma is tragic, because he can live only these extremes, and neither is viable. Either he is a dull object, attempting to suppress himself, or he is a manic subject, who will hear of no boundaries being attended to. Our mental health centers are full of these characters, who can only be managed by a huge control apparatus of antipsychotics, housing, close supervision, and a daily schedule of working and minimal socializing. Of course, they complain bitterly of being so confined, but prove its necessity by wild excursions when they are given some liberty.

The Ordinary Tale of the Chronic Mental Patient

It seems that it is sometimes possible to pose the dilemma of these two tragic horns to some of them and get them to rebel against their fate (White, 1989). Thus, "Is it necessary that you are either a dull prisoner, or, taking liberties, pull them into locking you up again? Is it conceivable you can enjoy yourself without someone summoning the police? Most people wouldn't think you can do it, but have to live in this miserable corner for the next fifty years. Are you interested in proving them wrong, or do you agree with them?"

Of course, it is absurd that a single speech of this sort would be enough, but it is the starting point of a map that actually works for some cases, so it is worth trying when we have patience to devote to the project and when the patient is not prone to violence. I for one would not attempt it with the likes of the Wolf Man, because he is so entrenched in his entitlement that he will be violent when he thinks he must surrender some of it. We have many patients like this, whom I leave well enough alone.

Behavioral Delay

If psychosis creates a delusional world apart, and delays the fall into pitiful prospects, many behaviors accomplish the same thing without the disadvantage of being labeled as psychotic. Thus, obsessive–compulsive (OCD) practices, phobias, hypochondriasis, borderline personality self-harm, anorexia and bulimia and obesity, alcohol and drug addictions, marital squabbling, Type-A-driven routines, and melancholia all provide endless rituals for marking time, keeping busy, and keeping other people busy so that the lack of a viable life is not reckoned. All of these rituals are capable of infinite elaboration that stabilizes them.

These rituals are one-dimensional, repeating the operation that makes the patient feel secure and recruiting a medical audience. Generally, they are treated by a program that obliges the patient simply to stop the ritual and endure the anxiety that ensues. These are all variations on what Marks (1987) calls exposure therapy.

The trouble with such directive treatment is twofold (Gustafson, in press a). The first problem is that the patient may not submit to it. The second is that if he does submit, he may end up free of the life-consuming ritual, and now be empty altogether, like a dry drunk.

This is why I prefer a two-dimensional framework for this one-dimensional elaboration. First, the richly joined system (Hoffman, 1975; Selvini-Palazzoli, 1980) has to be rudely and simply interrupted by one of these programs—anticompulsive, antieating, antidrinking, and so forth. Second, we need to look for what the patient prefers instead. Usually, there is a third alternative between ritual and emptiness, which has been hidden by these two horns of the delay dilemma.

A Case of a Has-Been

This middle-aged man looked eighty most of the time, while he was actually only fifty. He had had a very deprived background as a child and became a very wild and dissolute and yet adventurous youth. At thirty-five, he reformed and became an empty dry drunk. I saw him ten years later, complaining of depression, pointlessness, and suicidal ideas. The antialcoholism program had helped him to put a stop to his path of self-destruction but had found nothing to replace it.

Basically, he told me that he either dragged himself to work or stayed in bed. He was mostly very glum, yet he had flashes of retelling his old exploits. He could be entertaining, but this talent seemed to have only a past. When he wasn't busy, he felt like a rotten failure. There must be thirty million or more like him in America, those retired from former glory, in bureaucracies, professions, sports, the military, and so forth.

If I had been taken in by his account, I would have assumed only the two horns of his ceaseless dilemma, the former impossible and destructive glory, and the present pitiful and empty work. I made two other discoveries with him, because I was looking for what was left out of his self-portrait. One was that he loved crawling under the covers. It was an actual joy to him. It had its drawbacks, because so much time in bed made him stiff. The second was that he was a marvelous teacher at work, who came alive showing the younger bureaucrats how to do certain mysterious tricks with the computer. This made him feel worthwhile for short periods.

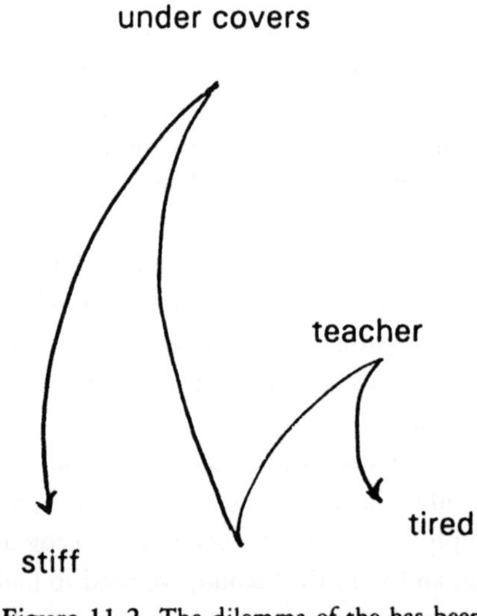

Figure 11.2. The dilemma of the has-been.

More than that I could not do for him. He was indeed a fallen man. The two unique outcomes, of his bedding down and of his teaching, could not be carried further. So his monthly sessions tended to be a litany of his glumness, his stiffness, and his barely hauling himself out of bed. In the middle of the hour would come a ray of light over a triumph, usually his teaching. At the end of the hour, the pain of the fall from the little triumph would be shared. That was all, and yet it was something. I helped him bear his trial of existence. Camus would have understood this kind of comfort.

Problem Saturation

A third kind of elaborate delay, besides psychosis and the behavioral rituals, is the practice of problem saturation (White, 1989). It overlaps with the behavioral rituals because so many of them, like anorexia, develop countless details to fix. Yet there are pure cases of everything being wrong, and little behavioral ritual at all, unless you want to call complaining, worrying, and fretting an inward ritual. I simply want to indicate that this third kind is also capable of infinite elaboration.

A Case of Living in a Brown Cloud

This lady in her sixties was tired out. She had become mother's replacement at age ten, and fifty years had taken their toll. Husbands, children, relatives, customers, doctors, salespeople—everyone had taken something from her and given little back. Everything that helped a little had a disadvantage. Antidepressants gave her more energy, but dried her out. Little vacations got her going, but made returning worse. Helping her daughters with their families was gratifying but exhausting. She was ambivalent about everything, and lived, as she put it, in a brown cloud.

She had the usual dilemma of delay: delaying her own desire and being worn out, versus having it and not being able to keep it up. Like the last case, she needed a doctor who could see what was left out of her story. What was missing was anything that had much blood flow. Her excursions did a little, but lacked force and were easily put out. I told her that she lacked an education about what pleased her. This education had been delayed sixty years! She just didn't know what she was keen about.

She replied that that made her very anxious. If she really found something that mattered, she'd be yanked away from it by all her obligations. Someone else would die, or some customer would go crazy, or something! I agreed it was entirely likely. The world would surely try to interrupt her, if she got on to something. She was older, and maybe she could be ready for them. I told her that Carol Bly (1981) wrote of middle-aged ladies in her town who were no longer willing to go to PTA, American Legion, quilting parties, and all that, but wanted to be left to their own devices. She was in plenty of company.

She surprised me by saying she'd always wanted a computer and to write, and

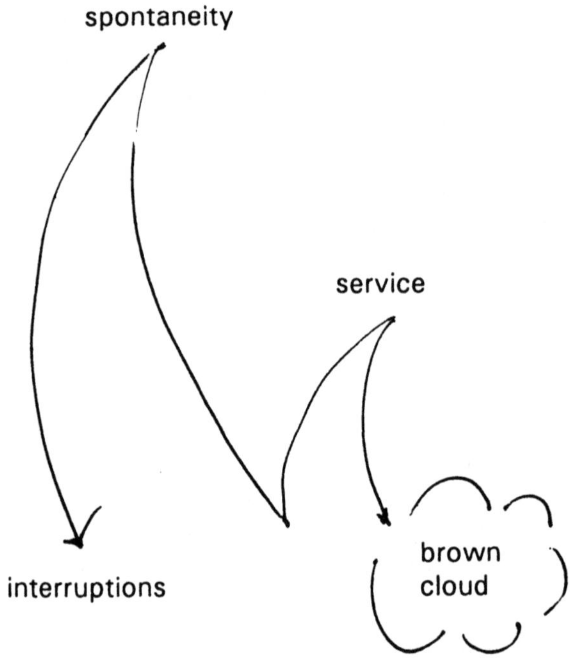

Figure 11.3. The dilemma of the brown cloud.

she was finally going to do it for herself. I replied that her education about herself was about to begin at last, and I even knew a class of writers with a fine teacher that might brighten her outlook a little. Of course, she put off doing it.

COMPLEX DELAY CONCERNS THE FALL OF MAN

The German Dilemma

I do not know why this is so, but German writers have shown a greater grasp of the fall of man, from the angels into utter baseness, than writers of any other country or language. Somehow, the German culture maintains like no other the loftiest ideals combined with the most bestial of practices. Perhaps this is what affords its writers the unparalleled opportunity of watching men fall through such a huge space.

The trouble with such a gap between ideal and actual is that it is very confusing to youth who love the ideal and come crashing against the actual. Often, there is a long and complex detour in coming to terms with beautiful dreams trying to play into a corrupt and entirely monetary world. This can take thirty or forty years to bend one's mind around, or one's soul.

This complex detour is the great subject of Goethe, Nietzsche, Kafka, Thomas Mann, and Freud himself. Therefore, I call it the German dilemma because these writers in German have characterized it most eloquently. Yet, we will track it into Russia, England, and Africa and into America as well. The German dilemma is precisely this: What saves a man's soul is his love of something beautiful, but what saves his enterprise is cold calculation of what will sell and, worse, even kill his competitors. It is truly a tragic dilemma. If he holds to his loyalty of his soul, he is ruined commercially. If he sells and kills for his enterprise, he loses his soul to the devil, like Faust himself.

The drama is apt to become macabre and strange. This is because the contradiction between soul and selling out is so unbearable that it cannot be faced. Lies become the chief practice of this gruesome and bald hypocrisy. As Orwell (1946) stated so clearly, language has two purposes. One is to reveal how things stand, and the other is to cover up how things stand. Thus, the Nazi doctors described by R. J. Lifton (1986) purport to purify the German State, while they murder like vicious rats. The contradiction is glossed over. Orwell (1946) caught it as follows:

> When one watches some tired hack on the platform mechanically repeating the familiar phrases—bestial atrocities, iron heel, bloodstained tyranny, free peoples of the world, stand shoulder to shoulder—one has the curious feeling that one is not watching a live human being but some sort of dummy: a feeling which suddenly becomes stronger at moments when the light catches the speaker's spectacles and turns them into blank discs which seem to have no eyes behind them. (p. 166)

It can take a youth a long detour before he pierces such lies to grasp this descent of man from the gods to the subhuman. Shakespeare's Hamlet never makes it. Kafka's youth in his story "The Judgement" never makes it, nor his man in "The Metamorphosis," nor any of his other heroes who die of broken hearts or are turned into insects to fit the base world. Nietzsche never makes it, ending up mad after a short lifetime of denouncing the *unter*- or under-man. Herman Hesse barely slips through, and his hero in *Magister Ludi* (1943/1970) has to flee the culture that purports to be spiritual and is merely a huge and empty hierarchy in a contest that has forgotten God as love altogether.

Freud's Irma Dream

Freud understood this struggle between high claims and base ambition in his own being. His first dream and the first dream ever analyzed, the Irma dream (see Chapter 13 for a full discussion of this dream), is about the fall of man in himself (Freud, 1900/1965). The gist of it is that he devoted himself to this patient, called Irma, but actually sacrificed her to the bizarre measures of his friend Fliess, who operated on her nose to solve her sexual problem and left a gauze pad behind so she bled profusely and continually for weeks after Fliess went back to Berlin and Freud was stuck with the disaster (Kuper and Stone, 1982). In the Irma dream, rounds with his doctor friends center on examination of Irma and exculpate Freud while blaming the other doctors (Erikson, 1954). Freud catches himself stooping very low. His own base ambition could hardly have been put in a colder light. It is the Faust in Freud.

Freud's Metapsychology

Curiously, Freud ends up putting baseness into the id inside man, and loftiness into the superego which is imported into man to civilize him. Now, there is truth in the need for the ego to bow to the superego, for the Faustian error is to be carried away like Freud in self-delight.

This premise of baseness inside sets up a long reconciliation with it, following in Freud's footsteps of his own analysis in psychoanalysis proper. It is a way, even a pilgrimage, for overcoming delay and even obfuscation about one's own Augustinian baseness. Certainly, it is a complex delay story that opposes two contradictory ideas that are very hard to reconcile, like the temptations of evil from within and subordination to God without.

Freud's Rat Man

The trouble with this psychoanalytic program to follow Freud is that it leaves half of the delay story intact, for baseness is to be found equally in the superego as representative of the culture. I have already discussed the case of the Rat Man in Chapter 8, so I only wish to remind the reader that the analysis of this character succeeds by translating his vision of German culture as a nightmare of rat activities, from gambling (*Speilratte*) to marriage (*Hieraten*). The man's love for Gisela is a childhood remnant that comes crashing against the culture's invitation to sell out altogether. In this exact sense, the superego is a huge rat, and the id is partly pure love.

The Plot of Complex Delay

I would prefer to say that the plot of complex delay is about taking the fall of man from God to subhuman, assuming that culture can be either base or lofty, yet there are ample arguments to suggest that its baseness is what needs facing by our patients.

English, American, African and Russian Variations

A child from a loving and strong family is apt to take a terrible fall leaving such a family for the commercial world. Thus, in Eliot's autobiographical novel *Middlemarch,* Dorothea imagines old Casuabon the scholar as her vital double, and finds him to be all dry rot. Thus, Henry Adams, the great-grandson of President John Adams, grandson of President John Quincy Adams, and son of Vice President and Ambassador to England in the Civil War Charles Adams, keeps looking for a beautiful eighteenth-century cosmos, and is disappointed by a world pulled to pieces by diverse interests that are merely commercial. Leon Wieseltier's introduction to *The Education of Henry Adams* summarizes the plot:

> The plot of these *Confessions* is not the struggle of soul against sin, but the struggle of the soul against dispersal, and nothing disperses the soul like society. Society distracts, it measures easily and rewards early, it rains purposes, it lasts forever, it legislates limits, it spurns inner voices. To live socially is to live an outer voice. (Adams, 1907/1961, p. xvii)

Dorothea takes a long time to recover her inner voice from this fall into dispersal, and Adams reaches sixty before he recovers his in his incredibly beautiful book, *Mont St. Michel and Chartres,* which, interestingly, is about the unity from 1150–1250 of Norman male militarism and female grace.

At minimum, the problem for the spirit is the one Adams sighted a hundred years ago for women who stood outside the commercial culture and seemed to lack any place of insertion:

> The American woman at her best . . . appeared as the result of a long series of discards, and her chief interest lay in what she had discarded. When closely watched, she seemed making a violent effort to follow the man. . . . The typical American man had his hand on a lever and his eye on a curve in his road; his living depended on keeping up an average speed of forty miles an hour, tending always to become sixty, eighty or a hundred, and he could not admit emotions, anxieties or subconscious distractions. (Adams, 1904/1986, p. 445)

The speedup of the machinery can be seen everywhere a hundred years later. Thus, an author drawn into selling his book by means of television promotions writes:

> Here is your job, a media expert has told me: to prove in 15 seconds that you are not a dud. This means having a brief, upbeat retort to the first question. . . . Speaking of open mouths, one's strongest impression is that the maw of media requires constant feeding. The author is a trace element in the diet. (Kramer, 1993)

This suction from the machinery, media in this instance, tends to pull in those with ambition and little else and stamps them out. It is a worldwide process—Japanese, African, Russian. Those who do not see it coming are drawn in willy-nilly, or left behind (Ba, 1980).

The Russian Invention in Reply to the Machinery, and a Case of the Humdrum

The Russians seemed to have got a start on all of us in making bureaucracy as dulling as possible so as to kill the soul. This is evident in the stories of Gogol and

Tolstoy during the mid- to late-nineteenth century and continues into the present with writers like Vosnesensky (1966) and Brodksy (1986). This long start taught some of them how to outlast the deadly danger in a subtle way. Most of us new to it think of flying away from it like de St. Exupery (1939) riding at dawn with bureaucrats in Toulouse:

> How many of us had they escorted through the rain on a journey from which there was no coming back? I heard them talking to one another in murmurs and whispers. They talked about illness, money, shabby domestic cares. Their talk painted the walls of the dismal prison in which these men had locked themselves up. And suddenly I had a vision of the face of destiny. Old bureaucrat, my comrade, it is not you who are to blame. No one helped you to escape. You, like a termite, built your peace by blocking up with cement every chink and cranny through which the light might pierce. You rolled yourself up into a ball in your genteel security, in security, in the stifling conventions of provincial life, raising a modest rampart against the winds and the tides and the stars. . . . Nobody has grasped you by the shoulders while there was still time. (p. 11)

The trouble with grasping people by the shoulders is that they still have got to earn a living. Few can fly like St. Exupery into wind, sand, and stars. The Russian trick is to do both at once, to be, as Vosnesensky (1966) wrote, in the World, but also in Antiworlds:

> The clerk Bukashkin is our neighbor.
> His face is grey as blotting paper.

This is a little tricky:

> But Anti-Bukashkin's dreams are the color
> Of blotting paper, and couldn't be duller.

No, the color visits in the middle of the night:

> Their ears are burning like a pair
> Of crimson butterflies, hovering there . . .

Of course, this won't count:

> . . . A distinguished lecturer lately told me,
> "Antiworlds are a total loss."

So, to put it very simply, my patient who has a technical job that becomes very humdrum also has very beautiful color in her dreams. Her Russian dilemma is quite like Vosnesensky's: If she becomes absorbed in the office, she feels terribly dull. If she becomes absorbed in daydreaming of her antiworlds, "Their ears burning like a pair of crimson butterflies, hovering there . . . ," she is apt to forget what her boss is telling her. It is indeed dangerous either way, and that is the structure of her dilemma every day.

I told her she had a long line of Russian predecessors and drew her a picture of the two slopes of her dilemma. She laughed and said my picture looked like Magritte.

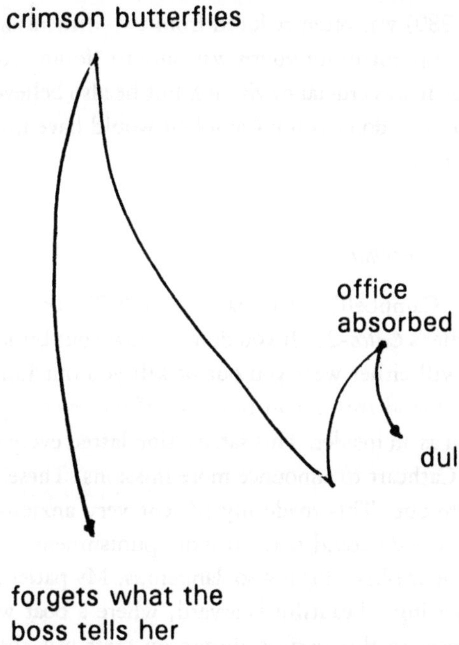

Figure 11.4. The dilemma of Humdrum.

More seriously, she went on to say she'd better start taking walks again to get her body moving, and she'd have to be careful also to pay attention, or she drops things and appears a klutz. I said, "Oh well, it is a double problem and there it is. Only a double description will see it." That appealed to her, artistically.

In my latest book (Gustafson, 1992), I described this case as A Case of Hidden Substantiality in the subjective realm. As a single description, it was perfectly true that she had a miraculous beauty that was blank in the objective realm. She had to go back to the bureaucracy. This double description of her dilemma maps the entire plot.

BRIEF AND LONG DETOURS IN COMPLEX DELAY

Perhaps the reader is familiar with Joseph Campbell from his extraordinary vitality in explaining the power of myth to Bill Moyers on public television in 1988. Here was an eighty-three-year-old man charged with the gods. Campbell understood perfectly well that possession by gods is electrical—that is, energizing—but also dangerous. You might descend into the underworld, leaving behind the academy, as Campbell himself did for a while, and never make it back. Heroes might lie with the goddess of the underworld for a week, and never get free of her grasp to bring back something beautiful.

Yet Campbell (1989) was often reduced from two dimensions to one, as if, to use his own phrase, the problem for youth was only to "follow your bliss." Like St. Exupery, he did believe it was crucial to vitality, but he also believed it could get you in a great deal of trouble. I don't think Campbell would have minded my restating his problem as a dilemma.

A Case of Campbell's Dilemma

It turns out that Campbell's dilemma is a catch-22 like Yossarian's, the protagonist in Joseph Heller's *Catch-22*. If you don't follow your bliss, you fly somebody else's missions. This will either wear you out or kill you outright, or at least drive you mad. My patient found this out in business. If you won a particular race, the higher-ups saluted you as an insider. This satisfaction lasted every so briefly, for there was always a Colonel Cathcart to announce more missions. These were dangerous. If you faltered, you were out. This made my patient very anxious, so he frantically drove himself until his body could take no more punishment.

If you do follow your bliss, this is also dangerous. My patient began to consider his, and dreamt of visiting a beautiful boatyard, where a boat was being made for him. The only weakness in this perfect aluminum craft was that it lacked a back door, and I was going to help him fit one to complete the boat. His associations to

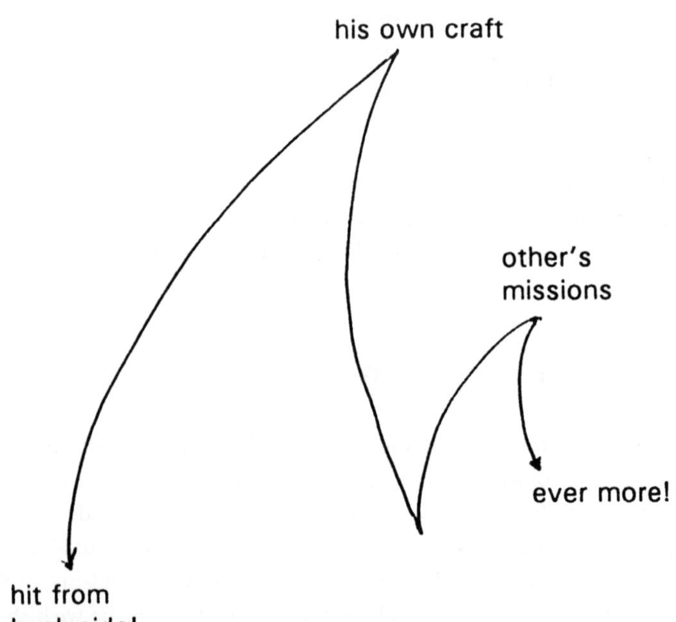

Figure 11.5. Campbell's dilemma.

this back door were about vulnerability from behind in trusting somebody. He had trusted several times before, with ruinous consequences. He had been badly misused.

In other words, this was a transference dream about easing up and sailing off on my couch. Would I ram him from behind like several others of a tyrannical nature? As he began to trust that I would not, he could not help noticing in his bliss that he became tyrannosaurus himself when somebody cut him off while he was driving to his session! Freud himself would have enjoyed this material confirming the Oedipus complex, the id, and the superego. Indeed, it was like one of his brief analyses, taking about thirty sessions, once a week for eight months.

We have gone on a little while longer and have not ended yet as I write, because he is enjoying getting a little more help with his dilemmas about his wife and his in-laws, his difficult partners in his business, and his extended family. Yet, they are all variations on Campbell's dilemma. If he goes along with them, denying his bliss, he sinks. If he pleases himself, following his bliss, he is going to have to get through rough weather with them.

In other words, their plans are to some extent perverse for his pleasure. His pleasure is perverse for their plans. There is always a fall to be taken, a sad finding for this Adam. After all, why should God throw him out for his curiosity? Man has been baffled by this for millennia, and so it is reasonable to me he should have a little longer to bend his mind around the rules of the Garden.

This is a very difficult passage for any man or woman, between the findings of inner delight and the findings of outer requirements. Alas, they are not the same. How do we get back and forth with the least harm? It helps to have absolute clarity and a very reliable map, or we are bewildered like Alice. Let us see when this can be accomplished briefly, and when it has to be a very long detour.

A Case of Enlightenment in Four Sessions

A young graduate student came to me with the routine complaint of having trouble finishing his thesis. Unlike many in this delay, he grasped immediately that the only way over the hump was to do what he had put off. He was a very rational man and responded to my logic.

He was also curious, and he responded to my interest in why he did the hardest thing last? I noted that I myself always did it first, so I could enjoy myself. Well, it turned out that his parents stuck to trouble like crazy in their own dark and stormy marriage, and my patient wanted no such irrationality. He would do what he pleased first, and, of course, that led to humps, like the end of his thesis left in front of him. All of this was simple mathematics.

I told him that his unconscious could picture the situation better than my diagram. I for one would like to see what it had to say. This intrigued him, being an inquisitive man. He got going on the necessary final job of the thesis and brought in a dream as well.

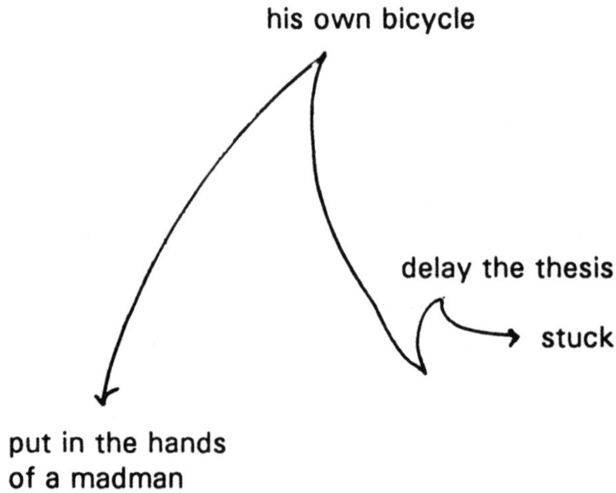

Figure 11.6. The dilemma of enlightenment.

In the dream he is at our local bus station, waiting to get out of town, when he meets a childhood friend who was literally insane and attacked people. The friend seems fine, and my patient catches him up on recent progress. It is time to go downstairs to catch the bus, but my patient has a bicycle to take along. He gives the old friend the bicycle to take down the elevator, while he takes the stairs. He runs into another old friend, who has succeeded in getting his thesis completed to get on with his life. This friend just walks through, as in a cameo appearance in a film. Then my patient wakes up in alarm, because his first friend and bicycle are nowhere in sight.

This turned out to be an elegant little map from his astute unconscious, for a man who had only trusted his conscious being. The map warned that he was foolishly trustful. This was a hell of a way to get out of town, to trust his bicycle to a madman just because he looked better. He would never get to ride his bicycle on vacation if he put it in bad hands. Of course, this madman was the patient himself, angry at the concluding job and just not taking care of business. He was being like his old friend, who just pulled his covers over his head. The dream gave him a caricature of himself as a warning.

He added as he went out the door that he drives like a madman just like his father. I told him it didn't surprise me. He was a Newtonian who believed in straight lines without impediment. Of course, his unconscious knew better but he was just learning. We had one a third session before he left, to help him practice a little more on interpreting dreams for himself. He was already very good, with help from reading Jung's (1933) "Dream Analysis in Its Practical Application," which I had given him after the first session, and with practice in the third session.

He happily brought in three dreams for his fourth and last session, now having completed his thesis and ready to go job interviewing. I will mention only one of the three, which pictured him lying with his previous and longstanding girlfriend in a mobile home in his parents' driveway. They were like stick figures lying side by side but head to foot, and foot to head. This seemed ridiculous to his mind of the Enlightenment. He could make nothing of it until I asked him what feeling came with the picture. He knew at once it was bitterness. She could be going with him now into his new search if they had not been so diametrically opposed about things like having children. Obviously, feeling carried great weight if he would attend to its gravity. I told him this was a beautiful algorithm of the heart (Bateson, 1972, p. 139; Pascal, 1662), that is, in showing how feeling has its own inexorable logic. He loved this idea, and left twice the man he had been.

A Case of Alice in Grave Danger

If my previous patient, still fancy free, did not heed his light and his dark minds, he would wind up in the inexorable ecology of the patient I describe next, who came twenty years later in a kind of iron swamp. These are much harder to get out of, much longer, and can be tragic. When you have ties, you cannot just dispense with them if leaving will topple lives. Yet the ties can bind so tightly that they give great misery.

Psychotherapists trained in the inner life do not understand this well enough as a rule. There are certain ecologies that set up cruel dilemmas. I am thinking of households that give ample room for the flourishing of willful offspring or spouses or even dogs, because no one is going to put his foot down. I am thinking of households that are cold as ice, or phony as officialdom, or those that are icy and fogged over by the polite veneer of wealth and manners, as Sullivan (1954, 1956) found in New York City; or those that cover savage opportunism with nutty idealism or office protocol. Finally, I am thinking of the strange academic self-centeredness that Lewis Carroll had to live with at Oxford. All of these bewilder children, like Alice, and tend to make them disturbed, if not downright psychotic or obsessive-compulsive.

The household of my sixty-five-year-old Alice was a cross between all of these things. It took her several years to notice that it bothered her at all, because she hardly knew her feelings existed. She was a thinker, in her specialized profession, who just was falling farther and farther behind in everything from A to Z—job, weight, housekeeping, and the like. She came for depression.

The first several years of her once-a-week treatment gradually introduced her absent self into the equation of her life, which privileged everything and everyone but herself. I was interested in what came ahead of what for her, and she began to clarify her preferences. She especially came to like finishing projects previously held up by lack of perfection. Essentially, I was confronting the simple mathematics of delay—that she could choose between perfection that piled things up, or adequacy that got them done. This broke through the enormous logjam.

It also threw us onto the inside surface, where she had been terrified as a child to show a self at all, and had survived by competence at grasping what other people needed from her. The dreams from this period were often throwbacks onto bleakness and terror, but like Lewis Carroll's Alice, she began to enjoy her own imagination. I have been asked why this case was a regular once-a-week long-term therapy. Simply because our routine steadied her in a ritual of celebration of a new self, which is not abandoned or intruded upon. She became a painter of her own dreams.

She had married in her mid-forties into a clan that was an improvement on her grim, poor, and even brutal childhood. They were fine and educated, and she was glad to take a back seat in deference to them, like Liza to Henry Higgins in *My Fair Lady.* However, as she began to come into her own in her painting, this deference in retrospect began to look more like submission and surrender of her interests. Also, as she began to show her talents, the good nature of Mr. Higgins proved very thin.

I can only mention three of a long series of night paintings in which she grappled with the confluence of her past, present, and future. One was of Mr. Higgins reading his *New York Times,* with just a rim of gold hair appearing over the top of the newspaper. Here she pictured what Henry saw of her from his perspective.

About a month later, she pictured herself from her own perspective, standing at a table of tripe with Henry's family and the whole world watching. She was repulsed by all these guts, but was expected to swallow it as a kind of ritual for the bride. She spat it out. She was embarrassed, but she could not take its bitterness.

Two weeks later she pictured herself fallen out of bed into a vat with broken

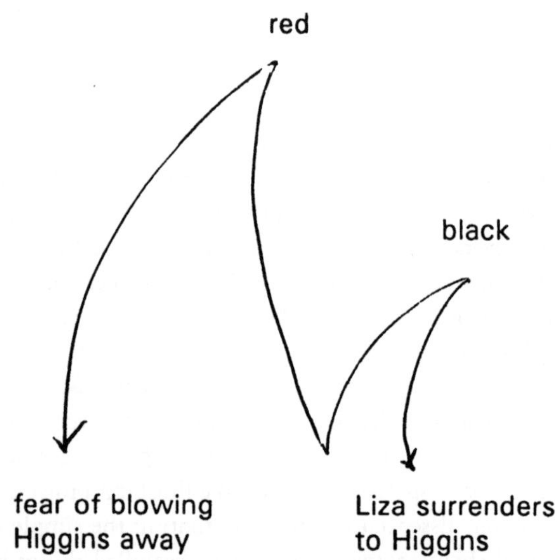

Figure 11.7. Alice's dangerous dilemma.

rings, full of salt tears. This vision alluded to *Judo* (a current movie), where a cruel patriarch is suspended in a vat and has to watch his beautiful wife married to the former servant who loves her. Instead, she put herself in the vat, because she really could not allow herself such passion at Henry's expense, even if she did obviously entertain such liberty.

Interestingly, she wore red this day, under her black suit. She laughed when I pointed out that she was apparently in mourning as in the suspected vat of broken rings and tears, but she also had a secret and red color like Judo. She was more loyal than she was revolutionary, and so the black was dominant, the red submerged.

This excerpt from her dream sequence shows the mighty struggle between her inner longings and her outer loyalty, which is far from resolved as I write. What is vital, however, is that her imagination can reach herself in her inside surface, and back out and across to the outside surface of where she fits into the Higgins family. She did not dare contemplate either when we began, so we needed a long detour to come up to these dangerous findings.

Like Alice, who had to go down a little hole to come to terms with the silly, arbitrary, and academic males and with the arbitrary and mad wives, she first found them extremely intimidating but now discovered they were but a pack of cards. She had to be careful, now that she could blow them away. She was too grateful and merciful to do that, so now she had a dilemma that would not resolve readily. This is the complex delay that hides a self, and hides the fall from the discovered self of night painting to the day self which could be dangerous in freeing itself up. It leaves her, even now, in a very painful dilemma, and so our work goes on.

Chapter 12

More Complex Passion

The ability to move widely and deeply in human affairs is sought by many writers, artists, ecologists, political leaders, or even psychotherapists. This freedom of movement is what I mean by a complex passion. Passion is from the Latin *passio,* to suffer. Oddly, the ability to suffer a wide variety of positions gives freedom of movement if one is not stuck in any given suffering. It is not easy to find a map for the trials of passion. Some patients come to us needing a mentor for this kind of life. I offer here what I think is needed.

COMPLEX PASSION

Perhaps I need to reiterate that a complex personality has at least two ideas. One idea fits him into the hierarchy he needs to climb in his specialty:

> Power in human societies is granted to leaders who *promise to maintain the traditional niches or even to expand them.* In this endeavor, two strategies are open to leaders that might be called further changes in the niche: Technical ingenuity, that produces more goods and services, or trade. When these eventually fail to satisfy, as they are bound to in populations of unchanging breeding strategy, only a single stratagem remains, that of taking land from other people by force. (Colinvaux, 1983, p. 4; my italics)

Thus, a neophyte has to position himself on a ladder of a traditional niche and defend its key idea by technical ingenuity or variation, by trade or circulation of its goods, or by going to war for getting it new territory. This is the path to power in business, medicine, or writing novels. This gives an individual range to move about and to be welcomed in sectors of society.

It confers no depth necessarily, for the professions all work by this formula of a single idea I have just described. Perhaps an example will make this obvious. In the publishing business, a company has a line of books that are its list. Since competitors encroach continually, the company must forever find new variations from its authors that will rewin the territory of readers. The readers are held by a formula they are comfortable with, say sex, violence, and drugs in murder mysteries. The clever contributor to this line of publishing has to stay within the formula, yet vary it to win the continual competition.

Depth comes from, by definition, that which is not on the surface. Since the surface of society is all mechanism—of the dynamo in the nineteenth century, of the cybernetic formula in the late twentieth century—the depth comes from that which is not of this world, from ideas, feeling, and visions that would be mysterious because they do not belong with ordinary success. They are a second idea, which comes from somewhere else. This somewhere else is the place of meaning, and meaning for us seems to be a matter of being part of a great and helpful force. This gives a sense of mission, of profound purpose.

Listen to St. Exupery (1939) in *Wind, Sand and Stars* describe how as a pilot shaving before take-off, he noticed a dragonfly sizzling on his lamp, guessed it had been driven hundreds of miles inland, and knew that only a terrible storm on the Sahara could do that and threaten his flight:

> What filled me with a barbaric joy was that I had understood a murmured monosyllable of this secret language, had sniffed the air and known what was coming, like one of those primitive men to whom the future is revealed in such faint rustlings; it was that I had been able to read the anger of the desert in the beating wings of a dragonfly. (p. 94)

This is what I mean by a complex personality: someone who gets around like a pilot in the world, but someone moved profoundly by reading the anger of the desert in the beating wings of a butterfly.

In admiring the complex passion of St. Exupery, I do not want to hold everyone to his standard, as if one had to live like him, fully or not at all. Indeed, it is entirely a matter of degree. One could live one hundred percent like him, or one percent, or any degree in between. In other words, anyone can have a complex project that can occupy any possible percentage of the personality.

A complex project (Sartre, in Laing and Cooper, 1964, p. 52) places one's present technique or strategy or form against the unknown, which is somewhat chaotic or random (Bateson, 1979), with the consequence that it continually evolves by collision, blunder, and new insight. This happens to my barber in his ongoing passion with how to hit a baseball; with a farmer I saw in family therapy in how he will plow this spring; with one of my friends in bringing up the big trout on the Escanaba River.

A simple project merely repeats because it is designed to repeat, and selected by a hierarchy for its control of a certain territory. If it has to invent variations, they are trivial in the sense that they can be predicted in advance, so there is no actual collision with the unknown and hence no surprise, let alone the barbaric joy of St. Exupery in understanding a murmured monosyllable of the secret language of the anger of the desert.

A life of complex passion is, thus, a matter of degree, in terms of how much one has it, in how many projects, and how much one is obliged to repeat the banal to keep the household going. This brings up the grave constraints of social class. Most people distinguish between upper, middle, and lower, as if higher were freer. Fussell (1983) persuades me that this is not actually so. He would divide the three classes into three sets of three, so that there is a lower lower, a middle lower, an upper lower, and so forth, the distinction being that the lower lower are completely controlled by supervision, and the middle lower mostly so, while the upper lower have more free will, because they cannot be supervised in their technical assignments, which call them at all hours and to all places.

If one of the latter advanced into the middle class as a lower-middle-class salesman, he would again be supervised rigidly. Middle middle has a little more room for free expression, for example, school teachers in their classrooms, while upper-middle-class artists and professors have only to report to God.

And further, the so-called advancement into the lower upper class involves being controlled again, because making money is a frantic activity that requires continually answering the telephone, smiling, showing up in correct places, and so forth, so it involves a loss of freedom, compared to the upper middle class.

It helps tremendously to have a skill—as St. Exupery had as an upper-middle-class pilot—to get free of the machinery of supervision, but this will not necessarily make it so. A second danger is that the professions generate what Foucault (1980) called "considered formulas," which control what is acceptable, printable, and showable in professional contexts and by extension, all of conscious life. The professor, hoping for approval, checks himself at every turn, even after he has tenure. He dreads being out. He becomes a variant of the considered formula of his field, 99 percent or 93 percent. Henry Adams (1907/1961) put it very well:

> No man, however strong, can serve ten years as schoolmaster, priest or Senator, and remain fit for anything else. All the dogmatic stations in life have the effect of fixing a certain stiffness of attitude forever, as if they mesmerized the subject. (p. 102)

A life that admits complex projects of discovery has to be positioned in the upper end of any of the three social classes or be confined to spare time. Furthermore, it is only possible for persons who have enough confidence to go against the considered formulae. This means being comfortable being on your own. Carol Gilligan (1990) suggests that it is easier for girls to be freer to be naturalists before ten, and Carol Bly (1981) that it is easier for women to take liberties after forty-five. In general, women have 5 to 10 percent more complexity than men because of their great prowess with those mysteries, children and reading, which makes them seem infinitely more profound.

There is yet a third condition for a complex besides time and confidence illustrated by the farcical movie *Clockwise,* starring John Cleese as the headmaster of an English school. Cleese parodies a man so driven by a formula for control by the clock that he surveys everyone from a control tower; no one escapes checking by the gaze of this big brother. He is about to receive an award as the best schoolmaster in England. As soon as he gets free of his own establishment, he becomes a creature of impulse, commandeering a girl-student to drive him, plowing across fields, stealing clothes, and so forth, until he arrives at the punctilious gathering of all the schoolmasters of England, where the police are waiting for him.

Thus, the break from the formula is so out of control that it arranges to be stopped. A related problem is that the break is so moving that it is hard to give it up, illustrated by another farcical movie from the sixties *Le Roi du Coeur* (The King of Hearts), starring Alan Bates. The break is created for a day in the life of a French town vacated by the Germans in World War I, because the occupants flee when the Resistance warns them the town will blow up at midnight, and the English thus fear to enter it. The mad get out of the lunatic asylum and take over the town, in lovely caprice, led by the King of Hearts, who is a Scotch pigeon expert sent into the town to investigate and who takes refuge in the asylum.

He is a marvelous, complex character who plays with the mad, with one eye on the clock, to save them all from annihilation at midnight. He is thus inserted into the machine-reality of men.

In the end, after the two armies destroy themselves in front of his royal box, he is obliged to go back to his post in the liberating army that soon arrives. He drops out, and drops off all his clothes, to reenter the asylum, because he cannot bear the life of military men. Thus, the movie ends. The King of Hearts has lived but a day, and must surrender or retreat.

If this were not reason enough to curtail the life of complex passion, there is one more consideration, which Henry Adams (1907/1961) called "mental inertia." It seems to be hard to think things over and sort through what is to be kept and what tossed out, even if we are asked to do it in our college essays. We do not learn to do it on our own, in journals, letters, or dreams, very often (Bly, 1981). Why not? Henry Adams (1907/1961) writes: "But nine minds in ten take polish passively; only the tenth sensibly reacts" (p. 302). Later, he revises it to one mind in two hundred (p. 314)! Why? I think the answer is purely Darwinian, in that it concerns natural selection. Children can keep journals and write poems and interpret Shakespeare amazingly, but the practice is not sustained in the face of selection by teen pressure, television, and the calling of the economic machinery. Liberal education tries to inculcate a counterpractice for the spirit, but the forces arrayed against it are a hundred times greater, and so the selection is natural.

Now, let us suppose that we have a character who has arranged to have a skill that is relatively free of supervision, the confidence to be alone and free of considered formulae, the ability to be free of being rounded up by the police for his transgressions, and a heart to love and yet retreat before the serious machinery, and, finally, a spirit to react freshly and see that it is inserted in the record. Let us suppose further that this character understands how he must come in low, to the groundlings as

Shakespeare did, to melodrama with his simple melodies as Verdi did in opera, to great strong cadences of harmonic melodrama as Vivaldi did. Like St. Exupery, he will deliver the mail while meditating on the dragonfly as his counterpoint. Now what are the troubles for such a complex and passionate personality? I will take this question in three stages. The first is that complex personalities are as prone as anyone to miss the great simplicities and go round and round in hellish circles, lacking recognition of the force involved.

THE FOUR PROPENSITIES

The four stories have their own captives, who live in one story predominantly. Someone who moves about more freely runs the great risk of falling into all four! This is why I call them the four propensities. Subservience, delay, overpowering, and basic fault stories have ancient names as propensities, namely, diffidence, evasion, greed, and mistrust. The old and territorial word for them is pitfalls (Peter Miller, personal communication). A complex being will fall into a pit like anybody else, unless he is alert to them.

Diffidence

Diffidence is difficulty in asking for what you need. Everyone is capable of it. Complex personalities seem not to have this trouble, as they have the aplomb to be themselves apart, but they usually have a nagging notion that they should be like everyone else. Thus, they can lose years of their lives going to dinner parties, school committees, and department meetings.

I once ran into one of our family doctors at a children's concert at the University Museum on a Sunday. He did not look well, shuffling his feet, eyes downcast, like somebody wishing to be on another planet. I said to him, "This is not *my* idea of a good time." He looked up, relieved, and said it wasn't his, either. I added, "Winnicott said ordinary social life is mildly depressing." At this, he positively started, laughed, and exclaimed how relieved he was that I had said this out loud. He hadn't known it was so, and thought it was his problem! He felt tremendously alive in his adventures as a doctor, and walked around a mildly depressed captive of society when he was off duty. This is typical.

One is not supposed to be negative about society. Can you imagine anyone reading this passage from St. Exupery (1939) out loud anywhere?

> There are two hundred million men in Europe whose existence has no meaning and who yearn to come alive. . . . Once it was believed that to bring these creatures to manhood it was enough to feed them, clothe them, and look to their everyday needs; but we see now that the result of this has been to turn out petty shopkeepers, village politicians, hollow technicians void of an inner life. (p. 219)

St. Exupery was discussing what drove European man into World War II. Perhaps this seems too far in the past to be relevant. Carol Bly (1981) wrote from rural Minnesota:

> This is the real death in our countryside, . . . this not approving of feeling. . . . They don't want to go out and beat up people, but they do have a very odd fascination for murders that can't possibly affect them. . . . The nonfeeling syndrome seems to work like this: (1) You repress the spontaneous feelings in life; (2) but spontaneous feelings are the source of enjoyment; so (3) enjoyment must be artificially applied from without (cute movies). (4) You repress your innate right to evaluate events and people, but (5) energy comes from making your own evaluations and acting on them, so (6) therefore your natural energy must be replaced by indifferent violence. (pp. 3–6)

Most of us are more diffident than Winnicott, St. Exupery, or Carol Bly, so we just go under in ordinary social life and blame ourselves. Nobody ever told us that human beings are finished when they do not have company in the actual difficulty of adventure. We were built for this, and nothing else will satisfy us.

Evasion

A second passive propensity is to evade something that will deteriorate unless taken care of or opposed vigorously. For example, many people are married to spouses or children who rant at them, and worse, for minor blunders. Their policy for handling this is to suffer the tantrum, apologize for the blunder, and wait for morning or however long it takes for the spouse or child to be good-natured again, if slightly apologetic.

This policy could not possibly be improved upon as a reward to keep intermittent terror going, and so it will flourish. If I pose this to such a patient, he or she will say that getting angry back creates havoc at once. I agree. It is a pointless alternative. Thus, many complex persons live as captives in their own houses, evading the implications of the hellish slope on which the terror gets worse with time.

A correlative and absolutely commonplace evasion in marriage and family life is to evade asking for what one needs. Everyone does it, to some extent, but complex people do it in their own way, which is typically to evade asking to be understood about what is most meaningful to them. As Jung (1925/1971) notes in "Marriage as a Psychological Relationship," complex persons tend to be married to simpler persons, and so have a range of interests in which the simpler partner will not be interested. Such conversational topics from the complex partner are soon apt to lead to a change of subject from the simpler partner, who naturally reverts to his or her own preferred topics. The conversation will shift to what the children did in school today, or to what the department did.

Without a clear policy to cope with this major difference in natural interests, the partnership will be hugely unsatisfying. Finding that it is further worsened by getting angry at the lack of interest in a wide range of subjects, the more complex partner stops bringing up anything that matters, drops into a shadow of having an adequate double, and evades the implications of the downhill course of the marriage, which will be dead soon enough.

Greed

The third and most active propensity I call greed, which seems to me to encompass all the overpowering urges known as the Seven Deadly Sins. These have been with us a long time, since the concept is Mithraic and "looked back (even) farther to Zoro-astrianism, which gave mystic significance to the number seven" (Turner, 1993, p. 36). Six of the seven are different active dimensions of greed, namely, pride, envy, anger, greed (in the sense of greed for wealth), ambition, and lust, while the seventh, sloth, is a passive propensity.

The Case of Dickens

Of course, everyone falls victim to these propensities, but, again, complex characters fall in their own way, usually by pretending to themselves that they are above such things. Look at the great Dickens (Rose, 1984, pp. 141–192), exemplary Victorian writer, father, and husband. He sincerely attempted to be a most eminent moralist of family life and succeeded, yet all the active six deadly sins ran away with him.

Why? He seemed to believe in his right to acquisition, and he seemed to think it innocent, and he seemed to have nothing much that opposed his voracious appetites. The more he fed the more they grew. Even his morality of the serene family household was eaten up by his appetite for more of it than he could manage: "It was as though his dependents increased geometrically and his resources only arithmetically" (Rose, 1984, p. 162). Of course this pace did in his wife. "She had given birth to ten children in sixteen years of marriage. . . . Living with one of the most energetic and high-spirited men in England, she was overwhelmed (p. 167). It was not only her. Everyone was.

> Dickens seemed to do in whomever he was with and then look down upon his companions, however humorously, for their inability to keep up with him. . . . Collins found it appalling. . . . And Forster, too, found all this charging up hills the expression of an impatience, impetuosity, and absence of inwardedness in Dickens. (p. 177)

So Dickens took to acting melodramas, which seemed to give him unlimited scope for being himself and getting everyone to listen: "He seemed to be living in a world with only one real person in it, himself" (p. 166). The most important sentence for me in this characterization of Dickens by Rose (1984) sits unobtrusively in the middle of a paragraph about his melodrama as an expression of human freedom and range: "For Shakespeare this image is counterbalanced by a sense of theatre as shadow-activity, an emblem of the vanity of human life" (p. 171). In *Antony and Cleopatra,* Shakespeare had already demonstrated the destruction of having nothing more than appetites. They eat up their world and end up empty.

All of us are seized with having to have things, status, money, prestige, partners, victories. Only if we can see them as this shadow-activity do we have much chance of resisting their vanity. However heavenly our purposes, we are apt to fall into having to have particular things, and that is our undoing, but hopefully not for too long at a spell. None of us escapes these fits.

Mistrust

I am tempted to say that mistrust is an abyss that returns perpetually for those who were failed in childhood. They have the propensity for mistrust like no one else, for any minor intrusion or abandonment drops them at once into a freefall that is terrifying (Balint, 1968; Gustafson, 1986, Chapter 8). They must always be on watch for its turns.

As a species in the modern world, we are all endangered, and complex personalities all the worse. The world of hierarchy seems to be interested only in its object, that of increase. No one can fail to notice its impersonality. In this sense, we are all intruded upon by its demands and abandoned by its market calculations. Increasingly, capital has learned to divest itself of unprofitable lines. Insofar as a personality has some second idea from which he is fertile in invention, the more painful will be his fall to the impersonality that rules everyone. He just falls from a greater height, which wounds him more deeply.

THE ITALIAN DILEMMA

How then are we to stay out of the two positions, paranoid and depressive, that classical theory predicts as altogether likely to keep capturing us? The paranoid position is a preoccupation that the world is out to harm us. The depressive position is a preoccupation that the world is indifferent to us (Balint, 1952). The first position is bitter, and the second is melancholy. Some people seem to be in both.

Of course, the world is out to harm us a great deal, and the world is indifferent to us a great deal, so how do we keep from *minding?* The answer is that we do not have to mind if we have places to go in our souls where we are free from harm and from indifference, and if we can readily decenter back to the world and our place in its hierarchy. A preoccupation with the destruction and indifference of the world signals one's inability to defend oneself from it, and so one is constantly or continually mindful so as to be ready for the next strike or the next neglect.

Simpler stances concerning the paranoid and depressive dilemmas simply comply with the hierarchy. I simply become subservient, delaying, or overpowering in my constant attitude (Gustafson, 1986, Chapter 2; Reich, 1933/1949), and lose track of my shadow soul altogether. At least, then, I more or less know my place, which keeps me from being shattered. My ten-year-old naturalist self is nowhere to be located, replaced by my adult self in the hierarchy. If there is no perspective from apart, and only one dimension, there is no comparison of this position of the real with the position of the ideal once dreamt of by the child.

Of course, it is there in shadow anyway, and longs to have its way and its say. This is why one-dimensional presentations always have two dimensions to consider, as in a dilemma, and this is why bitterness and despair are usually being reckoned, without the conscious knowledge of the person.

Complex stances are double at minimum, one for the world and one for the soul. Complex idealism is about having a world elsewhere. Complex detours are about coming down and back to a fallen world. Complex passion, our subject here in Chapter 12, is about making a mark in the world while staying free of its grip.

If an individual in a double or complex stance can do all three of these maneuvers, then he or she is going to be relatively free of bitterness and despair, overcoming the paranoid and depressive positions. He or she will move freely back and forth, between a world elsewhere and this commercial world, which cannot help being continually harsh and indifferent.

This free passage (Gustafson and Cooper, 1990, Chapter 7) is especially an Italian invention, responsive to the Italian dilemma. It is the dilemma of all modern heroes and heroines, but the Italian artists have the soundest grasp of the predicament, from Dante in literature, to Vivaldi and Verdi in music, to Fellini and Wertmuller in film. Selvini-Palazzoli has taken the benefit of this tradition to realize her own genius in psychotherapy.

The Italian dilemma is this. The world is one big machine, so you need to fit into the machinery to have a place. The trouble with qualifying to play a part, as a doctor, businessman, or secretary, is that you thus become a thing through which the machine stamps out its business: an overpowering, delaying, or subservient thing through which the force (see Weil's [1937–1940/1993] "The Iliad, or the Poem of Force" for its military equivalent) flows to transact the business of the day.

You keep your soul apart, in art, dream, and play. The trouble with this is that you will be disqualified if you show too much of this vitality, departing from the formula of your part. You are also apt to look for more company than what can be had fleetingly before your fellows must run back to their parts in the official apparatus.

The Italian dilemma is mastered only when you can play a part in the hierarchy without being swallowed up, only when you can play apart, without showing too much vitality or expecting too much company.

Dante first posed it in 1314, in the *Inferno* at the inception of the modern world, and at the close of the medieval world. From here, Dante takes us down into every variation, ever deeper, into the hell of being captured by worldly forces. He is saved only by inventing himself a double, who is Virgil, and then a second double, who is Beatrice. Virgil knows the stairway out of hell.

It is necessary to have a vision of heaven, and a stairway and a guide to it, apart from the world yet be ready for its assaults. This creates an antiphony as beautiful as in Vivaldi, or later in Verdi's Requiem, between the serene beauty of the "Tuba Mirum," and the crushing force of the "Dies Irae." Take away either half, and the art is vitiated and destroyed.

The double vision of heaven and hell continues in Italian art, currently in film, with Fellini and Wertmuller, who show the Madonna love and its ruin in the machinery of force, economics, and cruelty, as in *La Strada* or *Swept Away.* Many writers, like Tolstoy, Forster, and Agee, have tried to bend their minds around this fragility of heaven and the worldly victory of hell, been unable to stand it, and fell themselves to the tragedy (see also Calvino (1972) for a similar beautiful failure).

Selvini-Palazzoli (Selvini-Palazzoli *et al.*, 1989) inherited all of this, and kept her head clear. Her explorations with families taught her the requirements of Milan propriety. She must address their elaborate "concern" for one another in its precise idiom, or she would be disqualified, yet she must read the "imbroglios" or dirty games by which young people were elevated as allies of a losing parent, only to be dropped when it was no longer convenient to the status quo. In a way, the pretending was the reverse of the actual situation. They pretended beatific love while practicing diabolic destruction. She must go along with the first in order to catch them at the second. Only when she knew what they left out of their plotting could she reliably turn it up.

She herself suffers disqualification for her impolite findings, which offend the alliance for the mentally ill and establishment psychiatry that are determined to exculpate themselves and blame biology for the tragedies of schizophrenia. Tolstoy, Forster, and Agee all found this agonizing. Tolstoy (*War and Peace, Anna Karenina*) saw how the social spinning machine of society took nearly everyone down, but he hoped to stand apart like Levin and create schools for the peasants that could reverse the serfdom of Russia. E. M. Forster (*Passage to India, Howard's End*) believed in the beautiful connection of love, of the Schlegel sisters, of Dr. Aziz, but was obliged to show its tragedy when drawn into the manufacturing Wilcoxes and the Indian Empire. James Agee (*A Death in the Family*) witnessed the beauty of poor Southern families, ground into the dust by a cruel economy. Discoveries that help people become helpless when they offend the order of the economy.

Those who would pierce the logic of the Italian dilemma need to be doubly ready. First, they must expect the relentless selection of the bottom line by the mechanical-cybernetic-commerce without concern, while professing a great deal of concern. Medical students understand this perfectly, and come up with the answers expected by their professors, in place, on time, and in the right words of the definitions put before them. This is the overwhelming force, which makes man into a thing. Second, they must understand the enormous longing in the very same people for meaning that comes only from being a part of something helpful and profound, as St. Exupery (1939) puts before us more eloquently than anyone:

> When the wild duck or the wild geese migrate in their season, a strange tide rises in the territories over which they sweep. As if magnetized by the great triangular flight, the barnyard fowl leap a foot or two in the air and try to fly . . . into those hard little heads, till now filled with humble images of pools and worms and barnyards, there swims a sense of continental expanse, of the breadth of seas and the salt taste of the ocean wind. The duck totters to right and left in its wire enclosure, gripped by a sudden passion to perform the impossible and a sudden love whose object is a mystery. Even so is man overwhelmed by a mysterious presentiment of truth, so that he discovers the vanity of his bookkeeping and the emptiness of his domestic felicities. But he can never put a name to this sovereign truth. (pp. 212–213)

The hero of the Italian dilemma considers both of the great pulls, into the machinery and into heaven, and he also understands that the victory of the latter is transient because it is always pulled down by the march of the machinery. Only art puts it back up in the heavens, as Prospero explains to Ferdinand in Shakespeare's *The Tempest:*

> You do look, my son, in a moved sort,
> As if dismayed. Be cheerful, sir.
> Our revels now are ended. These our actors
> are melted into air, into thin air . . .
> And, like an insubstantial pageant faded,
> Leave not a rack behind.

It took Shakespeare himself enormous trouble and pain (Hughes, 1992) to reach this breakthrough, so it is surely something for complex passion to render unto Caesar what is Caesar's, and unto God what is God's (Matthew 22:21).

Henry Adams himself took sixty years to get this clear, always hoping like all the others that the world would build cathedrals like it did in the twelfth century, but finding, instead, it builds little political machines, forever dismantled and thus pitiful. In his *Mont Saint-Michel and Chartes,* he shows both the tension between the Love of the Virgin and the tramp of the Norman Conquest, and its suspension in the great cathedrals, and he demonstrates it as well in his own style of his book: "An artist, if good for anything, foresees what his public will see; and what his public will see is what he ought to have intended—the measure of his genius" (Adams, 1907/1961, p. 136). Thus, the hero has, at once, to sight god and to spell out something that the public will see, and applaud. The public will not do so for more than seconds, or minutes, but it will come back to it, forever, if rightly done. The machinery always pulls relentlessly, and most cannot spare much time before they turn back to its requirements. Thus, the medical students are moved by a beautiful interview but they absolutely must resume memorizing definitions from twelve different subjects. You would think the beauty never reached them. Count on beauty to be beheld ever so transiently, before its beholders rush back to their trains, in which they are terribly and *rightly* anxious to be included.

It will be someone like Emily Dickinson who will not run for the exits, because she knows they are hellish in their consequences. She will instead be taking her time:

> A Bird came down the Walk—
> He did not know I saw—
> He bit an Angleworm in halves
> And ate the fellow, raw . . .

The French, German, and Italian Dilemmas, and Three to Ten Dimensions

In general, the unconscious pictures itself to the left and the conscious to the right. The unconscious can bring into focus any region from left to right. The French

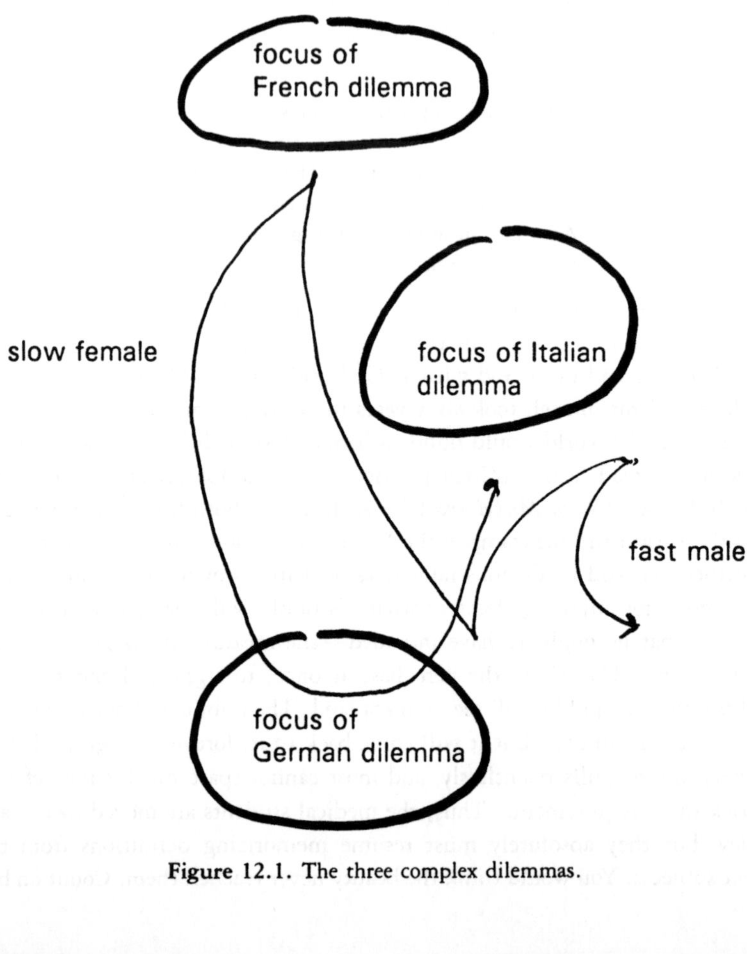

Figure 12.1. The three complex dilemmas.

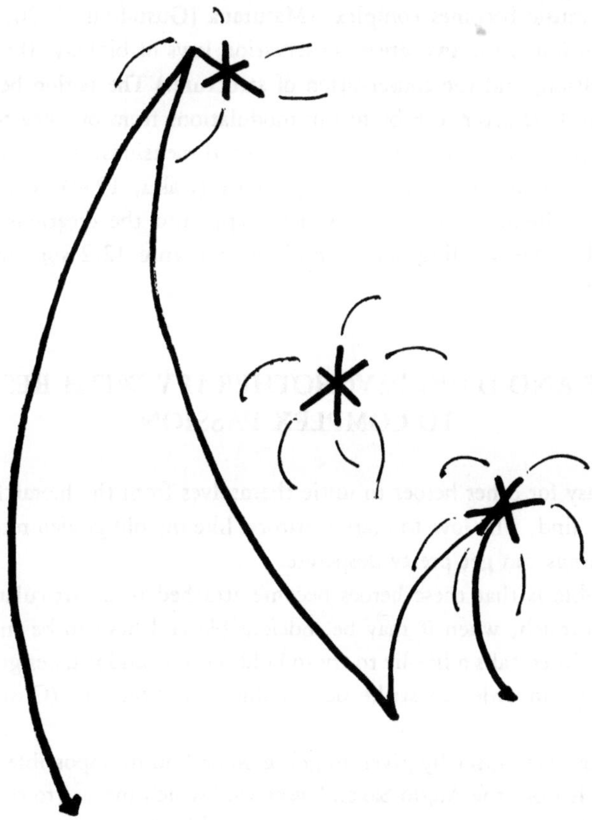

Figure 12.2. Hyperspace.

dilemma is the focus to the farthest left, that of the ideal, of the world elsewhere (Act I). The German dilemma is the focus in between, that of the fall from on high to the low (Act II). The Italian dilemma is the focus furthest to the right, that of the guile needed for reinsertion of fresh findings into the old regime (Act III).

The hero who will come through and persevere must master all three foci. For all heroes and heroines, Act I is the departure, Act II the discovery, Act III the return. Interestingly, the slow curve to the left for the slow, long, and beautiful development tends to be full of fertile female images. The pull to the right tends to be male and quick.

If three is the minimum number of foci (or strange attractors, in terms of chaos theory for a complex personality), many more are possible, as in polyphony, as in points of view in a novel, or as in perspectives in a painting. If there are huge forces pulling the personality into a binary form—to the right to accommodate the world, and to the left to accommodate its shadow preoccupation—both the outer attractor and the inner attractor can divide, like the melody and accompaniment can divide when simple music becomes complex. (Maturana [Gustafson, 1986, Chapter 17] calls these two forces the two great conservation laws of biology: the conservation of accommodation, and the conservation of structure.) The region between them, that of the third attractor, can be full of modulations from one key to another. In sum, three dimensions can complicate into ten dimensions, as Euclidean geometry developed through Riemann into hyperspace (Kaku, 1994). This takes us far beyond the requirements of brief psychotherapy into the creations of the most original minds. The whirling and crumpling in Figure 12.2 suggest dimensions beyond the three.

BRIEF AND LONG PSYCHOTHERAPY WITH RESPECT TO COMPLEX PASSION

It is not so easy for other heroes to untie themselves from the hierarchy, especially male heroes, I find, who love to mark territory, like my old golden retriever. When they can't, things can get pretty desperate.

The trouble is that these heroes become attached to a particular territory by marking it so much, when it may be indefensible and have to be surrendered. It becomes what Ibsen calls a life-lie to try to hold onto it, and it takes grace (Bateson, 1979) to let go in order to strike out in different directions (Gustafson, 1992, Chapter 12).

Smart guys are especially given to going on and on in impossible projects. The word "smart" is from the Anglo-Saxon "*smeortan,*" which means "to cause, or be the cause or seat of, a sharp poignant pain." Being capable of causing others to smart and get out of the way, smart guys get a foothold for themselves. The word "smart" has evolved toward a more laudatory, if ironic, meaning of "quick in learning, contriving, scheming." This quickness gives promise.

Often the promise is unfulfilled. This is where we are needed, because it is very hard for these fellows to back up. It hardly occurs to them. In the *Iliad,* Achilles cannot refrain from killing Hector, even when Hector begs for mercy. He plunges the Greeks forward.

Sometimes it is better to retreat, as Tolstoy's Kutuzov did into the Russian winter. Napoleon could not stop driving forward, and went too far and thus ruined his conquest. Retreating intelligently requires an eye for the long passage and a willingness to give up the short run. It helps to be able to distinguish the mission or campaign from particular battles. This is precisely what immature heroes lack. They confound the battle at hand with their very lives.

The help I lend these fellows is either brief or long. It is brief to extricate them from a particular losing battle. It is long to get them to be good counsel to themselves, and this may take a series of telling defeats and the passage of twenty or thirty years.

A Case of No One between Me and God

In Madison, many heroes come to scale the heights of academia. If you can get up there, and get tenure, there is no one between you and God. This is very pleasant. It turns very dark, however, when the prospect fades. Often not enough papers have been written. This leads to panic as the time to make it runs out.

I get many assistant professors who have begun to panic, like a particular man who was staying up writing until two in the morning and exhausting himself. Even so, he could not get the right number of papers completed. My job was to help him back down from the impossible climb, but that always involves a fall into the shad-

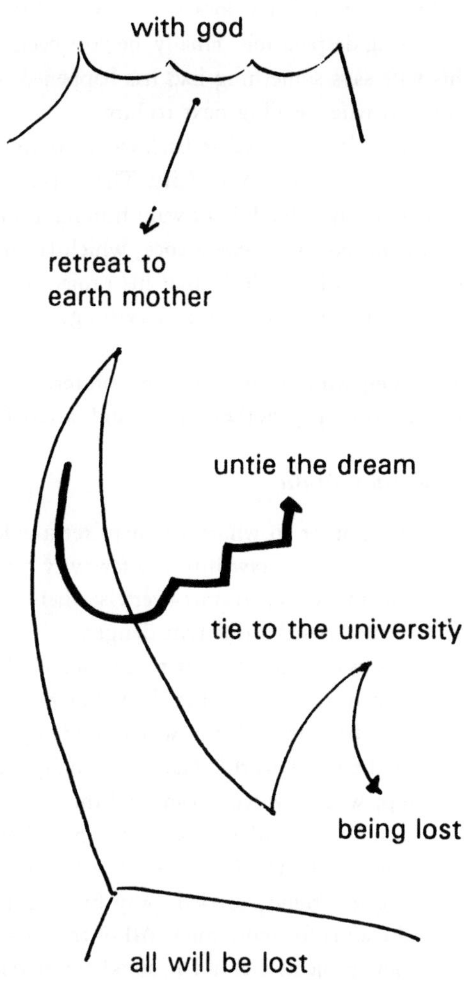

Figure 12.3. No one between me and God.

ows that is apt to be very disturbing. But only in that fertile darkness can a new project be conceived. This is an ancient idea, illuminated in the *Gilgamesh Epic* (2000 B.C.).

> Gilgamesh, in the heart of Uruk, will have seen you in dreams.
> Gilgamesh rises, speaks to Ninsun his mother to untie his dream.

The hero, having tied his dream to a particular territory—academia—has to untie it and retie it to some other territory. Untying the dream tends to drop him back into the childhood in which he conceived his dream. This is very painful.

The first dream told to me shows why going into dreaming is to be feared. I gave this man Jung's (1933) "Dream Interpretation in Its Practical Application" after our first session, whereupon he dreamt the following first dream to give to me.

He is in a very strange restaurant, which is in a labyrinth that reminds him of the university hospital where my office is located. His wife is missing. He looks into many rooms, with increasing desperation. Finally, he goes back into a filthy kitchen. There, a cousin of his wife says something bad has happened to her. He wakes up shouting, which wakes his wife sleeping next to him.

His associations to this dream converge back to his origins. The filthy kitchen takes him back to his poverty in New York City. The cousin of his wife takes him back to the severity of her family, who did not want him marrying in. His wife being missing leads him to her increasing independence, which is threatened if they have to leave Madison. In other words, he feels as if his project in the labyrinth of the university is being lost, and he dreads losing everything, especially his partner, in going down.

This is what I must help him brave, so that he can retie his dream of childhood to new territory. This is a brief psychotherapy through a terrifying transition.

A Case of Unearthly Russian Music

Sometimes, the earth mother to whom the hero returns for sustenance is not going to leave him but is going to draw him too far away by her seduction. This patient also had to leave the university to start over elsewhere. His first dream, after getting Jung's essay from me, posed a different danger.

He dreams his wife is asleep, but he has to get up. He finds he is in a glass apartment in a big city. There is water on the floor, but he cannot mop it up. He hears Russian piano music, a beautiful adagio, which suddenly stops. He is shocked. He feels this is proof that the spirit world exists. He finally sees himself as a child sitting on a toilet in camp, where everyone can see him.

His associations are to Woody Allen in a movie in a glass apartment, carried away by longings for a new female; to his mother, carried away by the water of the Holy Spirit; to his college girlfriend, carried away by Russian music and nearly ruining him in her grand claims for more men. All of this was about the danger of psychic inflation in his new project. Behind it stood the psychic deflation, in the exposure of his childhood.

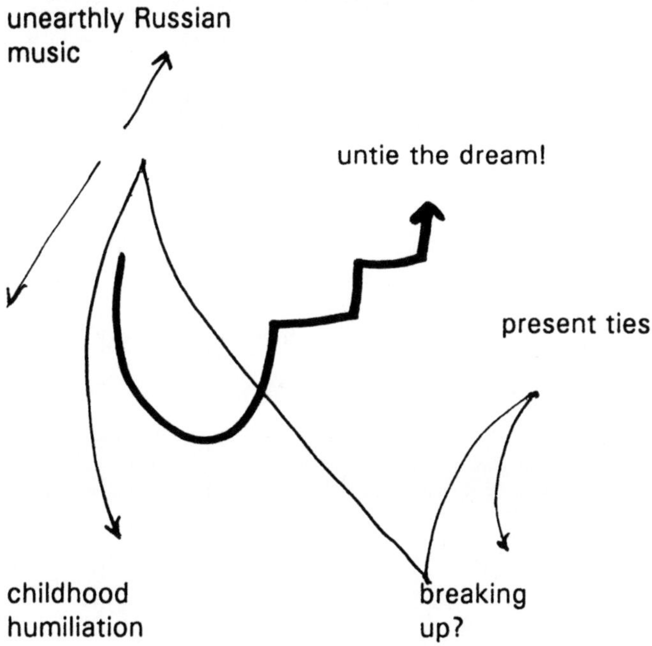

Figure 12.4. Unearthly Russian music.

We spent fifteen sessions on his transition, with the associations from his dream as the coordinates of his map. On the one hand, he could get carried away by his bigness. On the other hand, he could let himself be controlled like the little boy he once was. The passage lay in between.

The Royal Road of Psychotherapy

Freud's royal road of psychotherapy via dreams is usually thought of as long, as in a five-year psychoanalysis. It is not necessarily so, as illustrated by the previous two cases of transition by untying the dream from its locus.

I do think that a hero is not secured by a single victory. He only proves himself in the long run through a series of trials, some of which include necessary retreats. This is why I am teaching these fellows to untie their dream from its particular defeat, hoping they can carry on the practice for themselves in later circumstances. In this sense, Freud was absolutely right about the virtue of taking to a couch. It is a fine place to take a fall, to love the beauty of one's dream again, and to look for a new locus to play it out. It is an intelligent retreat (Peter Miller, personal communication).

Part III

Inner and Outer Worlds

While every twenty-four hours we all travel from our inner surfaces of dream to our outer insertion in the social world, and back again, we usually have great holes in our knowledge of this diurnal circuit. These gaps are the cause of dangerous oversights.

We begin from the inner surface of the psyche in dreams, where the gods speak to us for about two hours a night, but we hardly ever heed them. Jung (1963/1989) puts it most incisively:

> It seems almost incredible that though we receive signals from it every night, deciphering these communications seems too tedious for any but a very few people to be bothered with it. . . . We have obviously been so busy with the question of what we think that we entirely forget to ask what the unconscious psyche thinks about us. (pp. 93–94)

Freud opened the book of dreams for us in 1900 (Freud, 1900/1965), yet the restriction of the practice of dream interpretation in long-term psychoanalysis has had the effect of closing the book, except for the few. I believe this is a great error, for I find that the royal road of psychotherapy can be traversed in brief psychotherapy regularly. In Chapter 13, "Dream as an Individual Map of Dilemma," we look first at Freud's own Irma dream—the first dream ever richly analyzed in the modern world—for its marvelous clarity about Freud's dilemma in his own individual terms. We proceed from there to look at the two kinds of dreams that I distinguish in practice: punch dreams, which pack a simple punch from the unconscious concerning what the conscious is missing, and epic dreams, usually in three acts, which portray the soul's great journey into the world.

Chapter 14, "On Seeing the Social World Coming," is the opposite of Chapter 13 in that it looks outward rather than inward, with an eye attuned to the nature of the relevant structures of society. First of all, this means the structure of hierarchy in the late twentieth century, which is the structure of bureaucracy, with its considered formulae that create the boundary between insiders and outsiders. Second, this means attuning to amazement, the chief response to the actual activities of society, which precludes seeing them coming. Finally, and paradoxically, this means using the unconscious eye of dreams to augment the conscious and unamazed outward eye. Two eyes, conscious and unconscious, properly attuned give tremendous depth perception about the social world.

Chapter 15, "Ten Follow-up Evaluations and the Science of Brief Psychotherapy," is just that, namely, follow-ups I have conducted in the last year with ten cases. These are not meant to prove anything about my methods but rather to illustrate what I believe is worth looking for in conducting interviews one, two, three, or however many years after brief psychotherapy. My follow-up interviews, which are mostly videotaped, are studied for what Bateson called Learning I, II, and III. Learning I concerns the very situation complained about by the patient at the outset. Has he found a different way to handle it that reduces his array of symptoms (symptomatic and dynamic change in Malan's [1976a,b] terms). Learning II concerns the entire array of comparable situations to the one complained of. The question posed is the extent to which that patient has jumped, like Bateson's dolphin, to the entire class or series of related dilemmas, namely, not only at work, but in close relationships, in family, in society, etc. Learning III concerns the ability to continue Learning II beyond the original set or series or class of dilemmas that were a given, or the ability for continual transcendence. The idea is Hegelian. Any synthesis itself will harden into a new exoskeleton of dogma unless it is opposed by fresh currents from the unconscious. Learning III is the unusual capacity of the soul to resist the fixing of the conscious mind with the fresh currents of the oceanic unconscious. It is continual creation.

I am thus posing coordinates for follow-up that have little to do with "therapeutic factors," which have been the chief focus of investigations like those of Malan (1976a,b) in the 1970s and Strupp (Strupp and Binder, 1984) and Luborsky (Luborsky et al., 1988) in the 1980s. In the main line of modern social science, they attempt to isolate "outcome variables" and study their statistical drift under the supposed effect of "therapeutic factors." The linkages then are in terms of standard deviations in clouds of variables.

I am not opposed to this kind of distillery science, which creates a kind of whiskey out of a field of grain by breaking it down. We do learn something about the components of the grain, which do change with the methods of agriculture, but we lose the biological event itself by reducing its full faculties to something merely cognitive in faculty, or merely behavioral, or merely decisional, or merely emotional. I am interested in what can be achieved with the recognition of dilemma in all of its faculties, as a territory in which the patient lives for better or for worse.

Chapter 13

Dream as an Individual Map of Dilemma

For me, this is the most beautiful subject of all. It deserves an entire book. Much of value has been written starting from Freud's (1900/1965) *The Interpretation of Dreams*. I cannot review this history of previous contributions, here. I need instead to confine myself to a single topic concerning dreams, which is how they can be read as an individual map of dilemma in brief psychotherapy.

I choose to start from "An Analysis of a Specimen Dream," Part II of *The Interpretation of Dreams,* for many reasons, not only because it is the modern origin of dream work, not only for its beautiful clarity, but chiefly because it allows comparison with all the previous methods of dream interpretation. Many have tried their methods out on Freud's Specimen, which is called the Irma dream (Erikson, 1954; Kuper and Stone, 1982).

FREUD'S IRMA DREAM

Freud's preamble explains that the Irma of the dream was a patient who was only a partial success, from whom Freud had broken off for his summer recess, with Irma receiving a solution from Freud (1900/1965) "which she seemed unwilling to accept" (p. 138). A junior colleague and old friend of Freud, Otto, reported to Freud about her, after staying with her and her family at their country resort. "She's better, but not quite well." Freud blamed Otto's opinion on her relatives hostility to psychoanalysis, and the same night of Otto's report "wrote out

> Irma's case history, with the idea of giving it to Dr. M. (a common friend who was at that time the leading figure in our circle) in order to justify myself. That night (or more probably the next morning) I had the following dream, which I noted down immediately after waking."
>
> A large hall-numerous guests, whom we were receiving. Among them was

> Irma. I at once took her on one side, as though to answer her letter and to reproach her for not having accepted my "solution" yet. I said to her: "If you still get pains, it's really your own fault." She replied: "If you only knew what pains I've got in my throat and stomach and abdomen—it's choking me"—I was alarmed and looked at her. She looked pale and puffy. I thought to myself that after all I must be missing some organic trouble. I took her to the window and looked down her throat, and she showed some signs of recalcitrance, like women with artificial dentures. I thought to myself that there was really no need for her to do that. She then opened her mouth properly and on the right I found a big white patch; at another place I saw extensive whitish grey scabs upon some remarkably curly structures which were evidently modeled on the turbinal bones of the nose. I at once called to Dr. M., and he repeated the examination and confirmed it. . . . Dr. M. looked quite different from usual; he was very pale, he walked with a limp and his chin was clean-shaven. . . . My friend Otto was now standing beside her as well, and my friend Leopold was percussing through her bodice and saying: "She has a dull area low down on the left." He also indicated that a portion of the skin on the left shoulder was infiltrated. (I noticed this, just as he did, in spite of her dress). . . . M. said: "There's no doubt it's an infection, but no matter; dysentery will supervene and the toxin will be eliminated." . . . We were directly aware, too, of the origin of her infection. Not long before, when she was feeling unwell, my friend Otto had given her an injection of a preparation of propyl, propyls . . . propionic acid . . . trimethylamin (and I saw before the formula for this printed in heavy type). . . . Injections of that sort ought not to be made so thoughtlessly. . . . And probably the syringe had not been clean. (pp. 139–140)

Now, a very great deal has been said about this dream, starting with Freud himself, who emphasized his wish-fulfillment that he be exculpated from blame concerning this patient, continuing with Erikson's (1954) beautiful demonstration of its sensory modalities, and concluding with Kuper and Stone's (1982) proof concerning its dialectic argument about Freud's theory of sexual etiology of neurosis. All of this seems elucidating to me.

I choose to reserve my commentary to what is overlooked by them all, to which I am guided by my own map of the typical dilemma of an overpowering character like Freud. The gap in the commentary is expectable, if the theory of selective inattention is indeed correct.

Let us begin with what Freud sees in the dream: that he is driven to surpass all of his colleagues. This he knew he wished for. It drives him to be malicious. This he also graciously admitted. Yet, the alternative, or shadow slope, is to literally experience himself as the female, suffering Irma: "I noticed this, just as he did, in spite of her dress." As Erikson (1954) pointed out, he becomes Irma at this climax of the dream. "I saw at once that this was the rheumatism in my own shoulder if I sit up late into the night" (p. 46). The gap in the text is here. Freud (1900/1965) notes: "Frankly, I had no desire to penetrate more deeply at this point" (p. 146). The dream

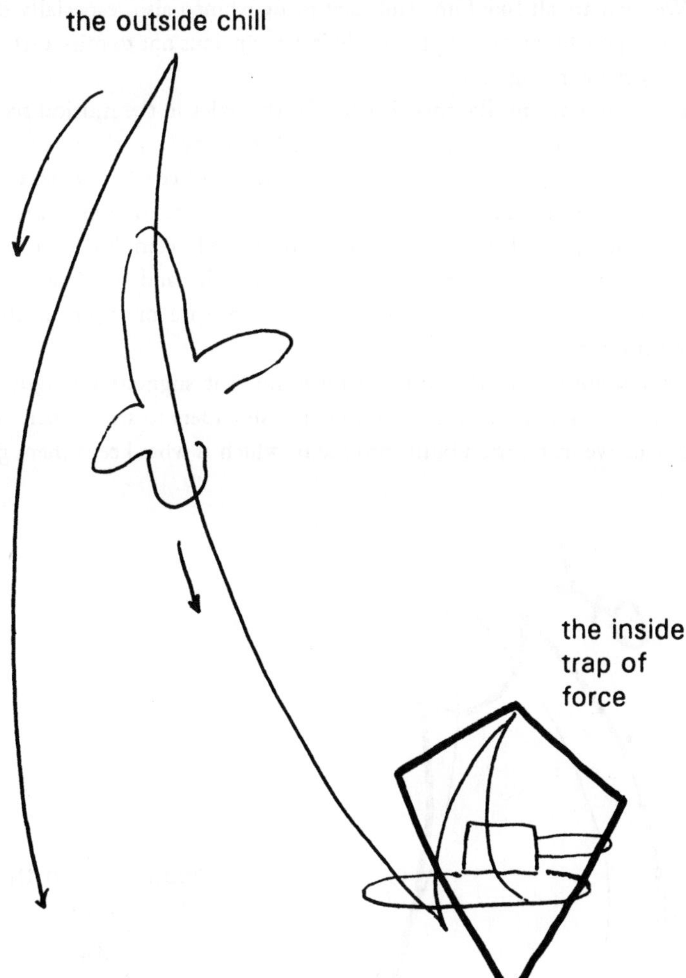

Figure 13.1. Force in Homer.

text shifts suddenly back to the verdict of the grand rounds led by Dr. M., which exonerates him and blames Otto, and Freud's analysis follows it.

Freud's seeing is all about his conscientiousness as a doctor. As he emphasizes, the dream is a "plea, for the dream was nothing else" (p. 152), for his standing as a doctor, which collects evidence from a huge array of sources for and against Freud's medical practice. The stakes are very high, and they concern his place in the medical hierarchy, which is precisely an increase pack. His fate with the male pack could range anywhere from leader to outcast. This makes a man extremely anxious to prove himself. We men are all like him, and now many women also, especially if we feel entitled to compete for favorable places. He is very anxious not to miss anything that would endanger his rising eminence.

When I hear a dream like this, I listen for the holes in the musical score, both in the dream text and in the patient's analysis of it. I have a patient experienced in dream work carry his analysis as far as he can and then notice what he has omitted to analyze. For working purposes, I assume the relevant score in Freud's dream is the plot of entitlement, which is overpowering and probably complex for a man of his power of creation. Freud's dream text has one big hole, and his dream analysis a second big hole, and both are critical to his fate, as they are for anyone in the grip of a plot of entitlement.

I do not write this in the spirit of criticism that suggests he ought to have known everything, for we truly stand on Freud's shoulders to see further. Also, the plots have selective inattention built into them, which is what keeps them going. A

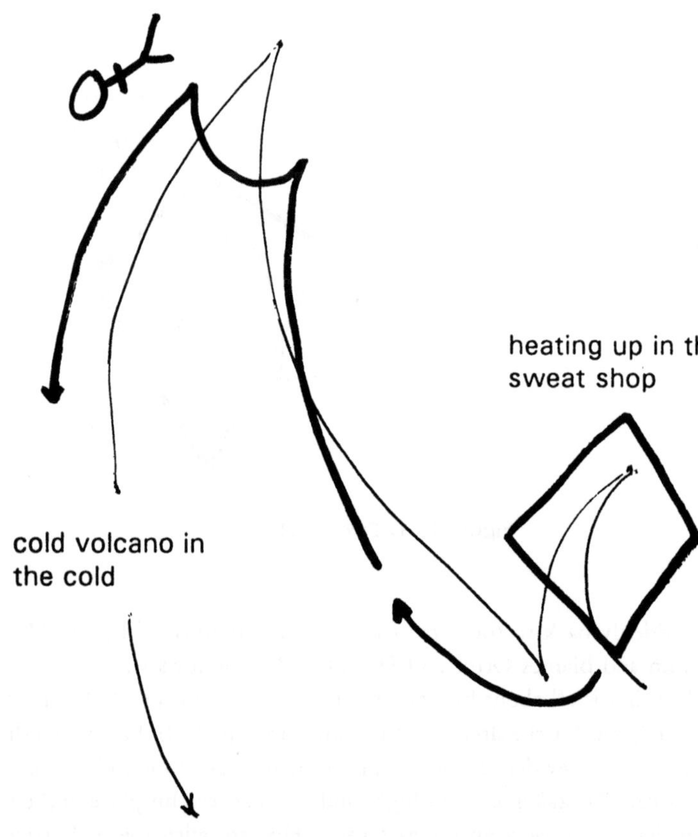

Figure 13.2. Hot and cold engines.

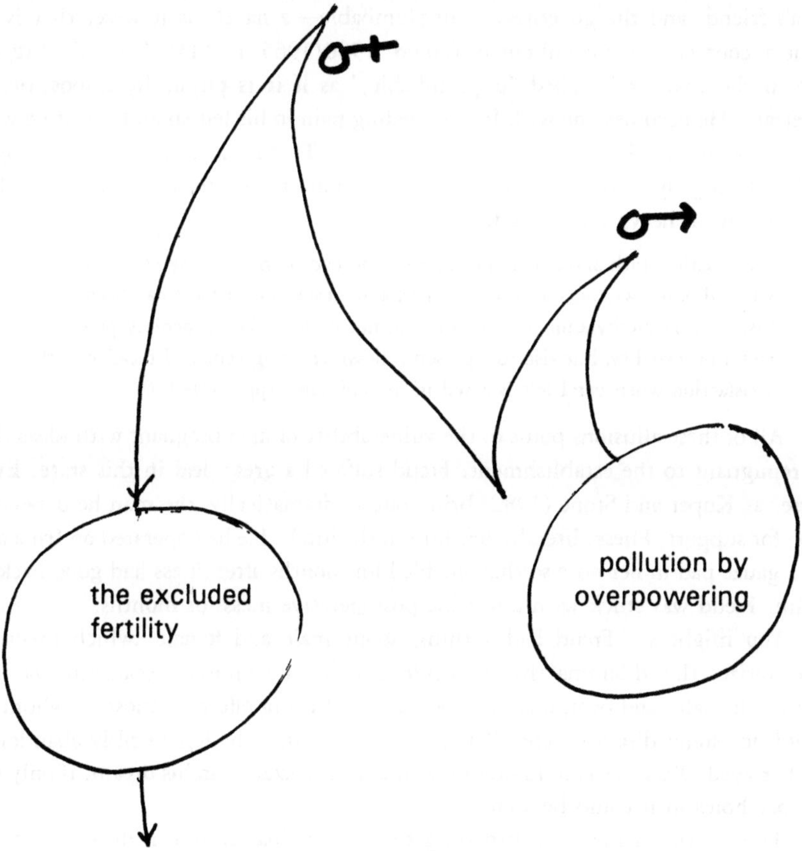

Figure 13.3. Freud's dilemma.

theory of free association to a dream will not find its holes. Freud could not have found them, given his premises about how to work them.

The hole in the text of the dream concerns the reactions of the characters ordered around, satirized, caricatured, and even falsely accused. None react, except for a brief recalcitrance from Irma, who opens up when Freud is displeased with her resistance. Heroes playing entitled parts overlook precisely this in those they dismiss. For the next forty years a long line of colleagues who had ideas different from Freud got exactly this dismissal. Freud was forever amazed, hurt, and then angered by their resistance to his vision, starting with Jung (Newton, 1979). It is fair to add that these colleagues tended to be equally egocentric and unjust to Freud.

The hole in the analysis of Freud's dream he himself notes. He leaves many hints, nevertheless, all of which are consistent with the shadow side of an overpowering plot of a powerful man. He pictures weakness as female, and runs from it. He even calls his thoughts about the three patients compared in the dream—Irma,

Irma's friend, and the governess—"unplumbable—a navel, as it were, that is its point of contact with the unknown" (Freud, 1900/1965, p. 143). Thus, the biggest hole in the analysis is called "unplumbable," as if it is physically impossible to penetrate. He becomes one with Irma—feeling pain in his left shoulder as if he were her—"invariably if I sit up late at night" (p. 146). That is precisely when he brought forth his progeny of discoveries. The culmination of the dream, of the word Trimethylamin in heavy type, alludes to

> conversation with another friend (Fliess) who had been for many years familiar with all of my writings during their period of gestation, just as I had been with his. . . . Trimethylamin was an allusion not only to the immensely powerful factor of sexuality, but also to a person (Fliess) whose agreement I recalled with satisfaction whenever I felt isolated in my opinions. (pp. 149–150)

All of these allusions point to the vulnerability of man pregnant with ideas that are repugnant to the establishment. Freud suffered a great deal in this state. Even worse, as Kuper and Stone (1982) bring out so dramatically, the man he depended upon for support, Fliess, literally left him in the lurch. He had operated on Irma and left a gauze pad in her nose so that she bled for months after Fliess had gone back to Berlin. Freud was stuck with a terrible postoperative mess for months.

You might say Freud had a thing about male and female, which precisely characterizes this dilemma that he could not face by himself because it was too painful. If male, and overpowering, he had a polluting effect on those in whom he would not suffer disagreement. If female, and original, he felt terribly abandoned and betrayed. This was Freud's dilemma, mapped so exactly in his dream, if only the two big holes in it could be seen.

This is what I mean by attending to selective inattention in dreams, a technique that will prove more powerful than Freud's method of dream interpretation by free association. The holes in the plot elude him. Only with a musical score of the relevant plot will the holes be seen and then made the chief subject of interest in the dream. That, in a few words, is my contribution on this subject, and that is how I am able to get powerful results on the royal road of brief psychotherapy.

PUNCH DREAMS

Sometimes doctors and patients new to dream work are daunted by big, epic dreams like Freud's Irma. All they have, they say, are little fragments. These, I say, are quite enough to start from. The key to them comes from Jung's observation (1933) that the unconscious mind sends us messages to compensate the conscious mind. So, if you know the conscious position, you can reckon the unconscious correction. It is as if the unconscious delivers a punch to unsettle the conscious assurance. So I call them punch dreams. (The term was invented by Vance Wilson [personal communication]. See The Case of the Missing Lion in my Introduction to the book for a beautiful punch dream.)

For example, whenever I tell a patient that it would be useful to get such messages, and give the patient Jung's (1933) essay "Dream Interpretation in Its Practical Application," the patient is likely to accede consciously while his unconscious corrects this by showing his dread. Thus, a man pictured himself peering out of his (dream) house while I paced up and down the sidewalk in front like the big bad wolf!

Another routine situation for a punch dream is an improvement in the relationship between patient and doctor. A resident had a patient who got comfort from his mother, but his father always became jealous and drove him out. In a few sessions, the patient began to get comfortable with the resident, and reported this dream. He was sitting in a classroom near a window, looking to a classmate on his right to tell him what was going on up front. The classmate explains that the teacher is pointing out the window to a frightening-looking man who is looking in the window right next to the patient!

The dream is an exact picture of the patient's dread of getting close in the classroom of psychotherapy, where he can hardly see anything himself and has to depend on his classmate the resident, who is looking to the teacher up front, myself, who sees a terrifying figure about to grab the patient. The resident did not know what to do with this dream when he got it, thinking the relationship was going so well and was shocked the next session to have the patient suddenly quit. The relationship was going very well consciously, which is exactly what terrified the patient unconsciously. Here was a typical situation with a schizoid patient, who stays out of peril by being half-in and half-out of relationships, who becomes engaged and endangered.

This dream was in black and white, which is pedestrian and diagrammatic and thus stark. Dreams in black and white, I find, indicate warnings about things in the world. Color dreams usually indicate warnings about gods, that is, forces larger than mortal life and more like the Olympians. For example, a patient concerned about a mentor dreamt of him as Sparky Anderson, baseball coach of the Detroit Tigers. Only the coach also looked like George Bush, and his Tigers jacket was blood red. This dream turned out to be an unconscious correction of the patient's conscious trust of his mentor, saying, unconsciously, that this man is consumed by ambition like the blood red of the Aztecs. He is on fire, like the sun. Do not underestimate the force that is consuming him!

A punch dream can be an entire brief psychotherapy when it balances a conscious position with an unconscious position, creating a unity of the two halves of the mind as follows.

A Case of a Two-Session Psychotherapy Settled by a Punch Dream

A very anxious woman came to me when her husband discovered her affair and insisted she break it off or he would leave her. She felt her dilemma was pulling her apart. If she gave up the affair to pacify her husband and keep the family together for

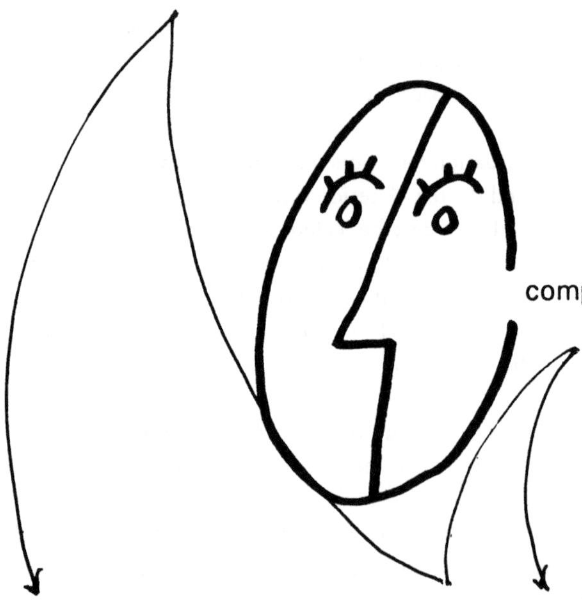

Figure 13.4. The riven mask of Klee on the horns of a dilemma.

her two sons, and for her own comfort, she would be repeating what she did at twenty-one, when she gave up her true love for this husband preferred by her parents. If she did not give it up, she would be torturing her husband. I summarized this painful dilemma in my letter after the first session and suggested that her dreams might help her decide what to do.

She came back a month later with a very interesting drawing by Paul Klee she had seen at the Museum of Art in Chicago, which showed a kind of mask, split in two, which she felt was hers. She also brought a very simple, but profound, punch dream, as follows. She dreamt of her husband's girlfriend, who committed suicide. She dreamt of the refrigerator in her mother's kitchen full of chocolate.

To make this hour short, her association to her husband's girlfriend was that she had submitted to him and allowed it to destroy her. This, in turn, reminded her of her aunt, who had allowed the same to happen to her. Her associations to the fridge were deep into her desolate childhood, where the chocolate saved her from going mad. She took the dream to mean that she had to keep the affair to keep from going mad and ending up dead. She would be secret about it, to keep from tormenting her husband. She only needed a little chocolate every once in a while, perhaps to remind her that it was there for her.

I wrote her, afterwards, to say she was in the dilemma of Anna Karenina and did not want the tragedy. Like Anna, she did not want to lose her family because of Karenin's anger. Like Anna, she did not want to lose her heart by surrendering to her husband's demand. She found herself a way to stay off the two horns. (See Figure 13.4; her drawing of the Klee mask fits between the horns!)

EPIC DREAMS

Epic dreams, like Freud's Irma dream, are indeed a big job, with many skills required of the doctor. Jung (1933) describes many of them in his "Dream Interpretation in Its Practical Application," which is the single best essay available. The gist of its practice is about how to take the dream text and translate it into a kind of individual vocabulary.

> To do this, we must keep as close as possible to the dream-images themselves. When a person has dreamed of a deal-table, little is accomplished by associating it with his writing-desk {free association} which is not made of deal [pine]. The dream refers expressly to a deal table. If at this point nothing occurs to the dreamer his hesitation signifies that a particular darkness surrounds the dream-image, and this is suspicious. We would expect him to have dozens of associations to a deal table, and when he cannot find a single one, this must have a meaning. In such cases we should return again and again to the image. I say to my patients: "Suppose I had no idea what the words 'deal table' mean. Describe this object and give me its history in such a way that I cannot fail to understand what sort of thing it is." We succeed in this way in establishing a good part of the context of that particular dream-image. When we have done this for all the images in the dream, we are ready for the venture of interpretation. (pp. 13–14)

This is Jung's "work up" of the raw dream, preparatory for translating it and contrasting to Freud's free association. Jung's method is determined to take the dream as a gift from the unconscious, by which it attempts to compensate for a conscious attitude that is unbalanced and thus dangerous.

I have found Jung's method to be the most sound, and I will show in what follows how I use it and how I have added certain technical measures.

A Case of Innocence Electrocuted

This case came to me when one of our residents told me she had been presented with a man's journal and didn't know what to do with it and asked if I would look at it. I did, noticed reference to difficult dreams, and told the resident I would be glad to see the patient with her in consultation. I spent about an hour and a quarter with them. As usual with me in consultations, I asked the resident to explain what they had accomplished and where they might be stuck.

Essentially, she told me they had a comfortable relationship, but the patient was stuck on destruction in dreams. He felt unduly preoccupied with the negative. She didn't know what to do with that to help him free himself.

The patient agreed, and went on to say that his ten years in the Army had been traumatic. He was now out, house-husbanding while his wife worked, and very anxious about his children getting caught up like he was in a very rough world. He wished they could be spared. His parents had stayed clear, his mother ruling their house with pure Catholic faith, his father being a woodchuck, off by himself in the country.

We are now about a half-hour into the interview. I felt I understood his conscious standpoint, so I could take, like Winnicott (1971b; Gustafson, 1986, Chapter 7), a drop off into his dream. I told him that he could not be trusting in God like his mother, nor be a woodchuck like his father, and his dreams must be all about that. He then pulled out his journal and read me the following dream, which I quote verbatim (utilizing the videotape to supply the text). My comments in parentheses.

> I had this dream about a girl named Sally. She was a girl I grew up with from first-grade through high school. And in the dream, Sally was strapped into this electric chair. (Oh, my word) And she was black.And Sally, of course is a white girl. I don't know why. I still knew it was her in the dream. It's a different kind of reality, or whatever. She was put in this chair by a guy who was wearing jeans and a flannel shirt. And I didn't know who he was. (I laugh here, as patient is wearing jeans and a flannel shirt.) Yeah, I wear them almost all the time, so it was strange, but I didn't know this person. (The costume was familiar . . .) but the face, I had no idea who it was in the dream. And my son, Peter, and a couple of other boys were watching him hook Sally up . . . they were putting this thing on her head . . . and strapping her arms down, and they were up there looking and stuff, and in the dream, Peter was getting too close, I was telling 'em to back up and give the man room to work. And I remember people coming in, and this was in our old high school gymnasium. I recognize it because it was an old, very familiar building. And people were coming in to watch the electrocution and they were brushing heavy snow off themselves and mumbling to themselves and going up into the stands and . . . the guy in the flannel shirt kept taking smoke breaks, so the people were grumbling about why the thing wasn't getting underway, and why it hadn't started yet and this kind of thing. And then finally, he was ready to electrocute her, and Peter asked if he could help. And the man rubs his head, and that kind of thing, and then the phone rang. And it was Sally's Mom, who said Sally doesn't need to be electrocuted anymore, because it is snowing heavily, and everybody should go home. (I laugh.) And I don't know why I answer the phone. There were all these people there, but I answer the phone. It was kind of a weird thing. So . . . I help the guy unhook Sally. And Peter asks if he could go outside and start the car. So I give him the keys and he went out . . . and . . . I went out afterwards, after we were all done I went out to find him and I saw . . . it was blizzarding like crazy . . . and I saw one set of headlights . . . and in the dream, I didn't even think those might be Peter . . . or anything. I couldn't find Peter, so I ran around yelling for Peter in the snow and then I woke up. It was a nightmare. I woke up really (shaking.) Yeah. (Not able to find him.) Right. (In the snow.) Right. (So it's very frightening in the end.)

Although I have his conscious standpoint clear in the present, I also want it from the night before the dream, so I ask him about it, and he consults his journal to tell me that he and his wife and extended family had gone dancing and had fun, which had been missing for many years of the Army life.

He is very shaky after telling me the dream. I ask him about it, and he says he would rather not be so negative and just have fun, which would be better for his family. I reply that it seems he *is* negative, which we had better see about. In other words, his conscious standpoint is that the negative is bad, and hard for his family because he is so often down, and therefore it ought to be purged. His unconscious standpoint about the negative now remains to be discovered.

Now we begin our work-up of translating the vocabulary of the dream, starting with his remark that he is but twelve or thirteen in the dream. I say, yes, still innocent, and he looks upset. When feeling surfaces strongly at any point in our analysis, I ride with it. He says it is the last time he had fun. He misses his childhood. I say, we are back before the fall. He tells me about Sally, his pal in those days.

I now ask about the electrocution. This leads to a terrible memory. As Jung suggests, the key is to know what this subject means to him in particular in the history of his life. The classical, Freudian way to ask for that context is to say: "What comes to mind about electrocution?" For me, this way of asking often brings up too much to think about. I find I get more of the individual context by asking: "Where does electrocution take you?" If that takes us nowhere, I am apt to ask: "What is your feeling about electrocution?" This failing to generate anything, I am apt to explain that electrocution has a meaning for him, in particular, so I would like to know where, when, and how he has run into electrocution.

Here, his feeling was horrible, and took him back to being nineteen, working on a crew fixing power lines. A kid next to him went up an aluminum ladder that touched a live line, and literally blew the kid up. My patient was terribly shaken. I responded that this ought never to have happened.

The blackness of Sally in the dream took him back to the Army where racial hatred was a daily trial. He recalled his fright going to the shower, having to carry a baseball bat to defend himself from possible assault. Again, he was shaken. I responded that this was another one of those things that should not be.

Already, great emotion was moving in him in opposing currents, between white innocence and the terrible fall into evil, which, for him, is black. Afro-American readers have always known about the white unconscious, which is perfectly obvious in eighteenth- and nineteenth-century novels in which white heroines are good and black heroines are thrilling but evil. Interestingly, this patient reverses the field by showing the white guy in flannel as evil to the black girl in what Arendt (1963) would call the banality of evil. Rather than wait until we have translated each element of the dream, I am more likely to sound what the dream it seems to mean as we go along. I don't interpret hard and fast at all, but I am making soundings. I feel I know where the unconscious is going. I sense it, and the patient's growing intensity suggests I am headed in the right direction. All three of the terms translated—being twelve, electrocution, and black Sally—are very contrary to present reality, which means they are likely to be laden with meaning (Freud, 1900/1965). This was a dream calling out to be unburdened.

The fourth element I asked him about was the regular guy who is the executioner. This part amazed him, and he didn't have much to say about it until I said, blandly, "Regular guys can do terrible things." This seemed to take him far away. I am quite convinced, like Winnicott (1971; Gustafson, 1986, Chapter 7), that patients will not go to the most unbearable experiences without company. My intonation of the plot gave this company.

He remembered working in a plant where he supplied a conveyor belt with materials taken up and dropped into a vat where they were chopped to pieces. When the belt got stuck, he yelled at the operator to shut it off, and he went up the belt to unstick it. The guy turned the belt back on, sending him over the top, and almost into the vat with the huge scissors, except that he caught himself on the bar in the middle and spun around, barely saving himself. Somehow, the guy heard him yelling and stopped the belt, but when he crawled down, he fell upon the guy berserk with rage.

I responded, "He was awfully careless with your life." He replied, "He wasn't thinking," and now began to get shaky and flustered, his neck reddening. We seemed to be in a tunnel, going from one unbearable experience to another, but I did not know where we were going to come out. We had passed back from the facade of the executioner into the depth of the dream house of his near execution and now penetrated even farther back into his unconscious.

Sensing he was traveling far back, knowing he needed my company, I sounded for him again, telling him that we were going into the evil of regular guys and toward the problem of protecting his son, Peter (following the text of the dream). This must have been enough for him to summon the courage to tell me the following story. He had been in a very beautiful place in the Pacific snorkeling with his buddies off duty. A typhoon came up so fast that they barely got back to the beach in time to fly to the emergency bunker. The storm hit. He forgot to tell anybody that there were two other guys out sailing, and they were never seen again. Now his shakiness turned to tears. He felt that he too had been careless with lives.

We dwelt with this awhile. He had carried around his self-blame for this for many years. After a while, he seemed to have gotten it out, and asked, "Well, so what?"

Even though we were only halfway through the dream, I could summarize what we seemed to have as a correction from his unconscious. While he consciously believed it was better to purge the negative, his unconscious felt that he had to remember carelessness with lives at all cost! He couldn't trust God to take care of things, like his mother did, nor bury his head like the woodchuck his father was. He had children going into the world who needed looking out for. This seemed like a revelation to him. We were past our allotted hour, so I proposed we just run over another ten minutes and finish up. "What about Sally's mother calling off the whole thing? It seems like comic relief." "Well, that was easy," he said. "I just wish these things didn't happen." "And the headlights in the snow?" "Well, I got up from the dream and went straight to Peter's room to make sure he was all right."

We had to finish. I said, with considerable feeling myself as a fellow father, "You'd better keep an eye on that boy." Of course, this was emotional shorthand for the huge subject of preparing an innocent boy for an electrocuting world.

A Few Further Technical Remarks

Going through this dream with this man was one of the most moving experiences of my life as a doctor. I tell it not because dream work often gets to this level of

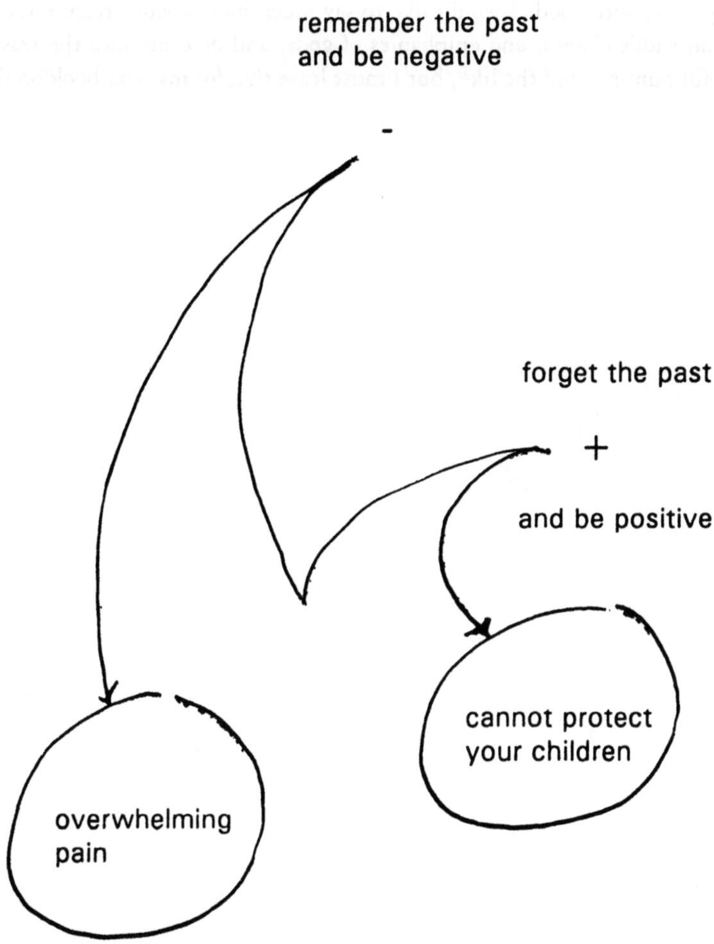

Figure 13.5. A case of innocence electrocuted.

intensity, but because I hope it will be unforgettable for the reader. I hope the reader understands my meaning about what it is to work up a dream so that the patient gets an extraordinary and individual map of his dilemma directly from his own unconscious. Here is this patient's dilemma: If he is consciously positive, he is in danger of carelessness with lives. If he is negative, he cannot find his way back to the delightful innocence of childhood that his family also needs from him. It is a balance to work out, between those two dangerous slopes.

If I had had the opportunity to go on with this man as my patient, I would have been tremendously interested in the sequence of dreams that followed this one. I would have him do what work he could translating each element, and summarizing, and wait for my turn to take up the elements he overlooked in his selective inattention, which holds, invariably, the unbearable aspects that need my eye and my company to be withstood. I would like to say much more about dream screens, and tempo and sudden flows, and epiphanies of gods, and descents into the wasteland, and helpful numina, and the like, but I must leave that for my next book on dreams.

Chapter 14

On Seeing the Social World Coming

All the books ever written have something to say, on some topic, special or general, about how the world works. After all, we might need to know about termites eating up our house, or we might need to know about the zodiac, fascinating our teenagers. It might seem fantastic at first thought to reduce all of the books on the world to one chapter.

I propose to do this, because I find my patients keep colliding with the same structure over and over again. They have made the selection for me. This must be crucial knowledge. For lack of it people become miserable, and often are ruined.

What is this structure that is overlooked? It is the social hierarchy, which is an extremely forceful machine (Levi-Strauss in Charbonnier, 1969). We are selected either to fit into it or be cast out. Why and how would my patients overlook something with such overwhelming consequences? After all, dogs know how to get along in a dog pack. Why and how would we be any different?

The reason is that humans start from packs called families, which are often refuges from the larger packs called society. It is commonplace for immature humans to fit the family pack, but not the larger packs of the neighborhood, the school, jobs, and so forth.

Some families fit their offspring very neatly into the world. Thus, bankers in France know how to get their children ready for banking, and academics know how to get their children ready for academia (Bourdieu, 1984). While one fitting into the economic machinery may be considered a success, the experience is not necessarily meaningful.

There are two great and terrible outcomes, with respect to the economic packs that are the main structure of our world. One is to be left out of them. The other is to be confined within them. My patients miss these things because their families miss them and because they never got a compensatory education. I am often called upon to provide it in psychotherapy.

JUNG'S DILEMMA

This education can be summarized in terms of grasping the two great dangers of the social hierarchy as the horns of a dilemma. I would like to call it Jung's dilemma, because I think he posed it to his patients better than any other writer in our field (Jung, 1971a). In his terms, the patient is likely to be impaled by the part he plays in society, which Jung called the persona. This mask becomes all there is to the personality.

Alternatively, the patient becomes an outsider, where he is likely to be taken over by primordial images that run away with him, so that he suffers the psychic inflation of feeling himself to be a god, or the psychic deflation of being a nobody.

Jung's dilemma is played out in grave terms by all of us in three distinct domains: work, society, and love. We take each in its turn.

Work

To get paid for your skill, you have to have a position in the market where that skill is sought. Mostly, you get a position by moving up a ladder that tests your qualifications. Often, when there are many qualifiers, the person with connections gets the nod. All of this may seem extremely obvious, but many miss the obvious. I see patients with great skill in art or in psychotherapy, who belong to no guild or profession and get no audience or clients whatsoever. I see patients who hope to be doctors, but cannot undergo the first step of the ladder in introductory chemistry. I see patients who hope to be musicians or scientists, but imagine doing it strictly on skill, without the help of high-placed mentors.

Conversely, those who get into the hierarchies of teaching, of academia, or of medicine regularly find themselves trapped. I have patients in education, who are astonished that their superiors do not back them in their dealings with impossible parents. I have patients in academia, who are shocked that their superiors merely want their research data. I have patients in medicine, who are flabbergasted that they are given more and more patients to take care of but receive less help. All of this may seem extremely obvious, but many miss the obvious. They expect a working world that cares for more than numbers.

In other words, all of these patients look at the working world with a big hole in their visual field, which is created by a mistaken idea. The outsiders propose to get ahead, while ignoring the strict rules of ascent into the hierarchies. The insiders propose to enjoy their positions in the hierarchies, while ignoring what maintains them in place. It really is all so impersonal, and we do not want to come to terms with the machinery.

Slightly more complex cases involve trouble as an insider *and* as an outsider.

A Case of Depression in the First Week of School, Revisited

I described this case in Chapter 7 as a classical delay story, and I now return to it to show its significance as a typical collision with the economic machinery. The reader may remember that this young woman took a mighty plunge from a free summer of bicycling in Indiana, to surrendering to a course that would waste her time, taught by an old man (professor). She went from light to utter darkness, as if turning herself over to the system to be put in a dungeon. She went from an ephemeral butterfly spirit to larval torpor.

As it turned out, I looked for and found two big holes in the story. The first was on the inner surface. I just did not believe she had no feelings about having her time wasted for an entire semester. This led into her rage, and her guilt about her rage. This took us back to her father. After all, it was his premise, taken on by her, that you had to earn a living by surrendering to whatever the company asked of you! It was his jumping on her for taking liberty that had been the most painful episode of her existence.

She had tried very hard to be like him, out of love and fear, which is what we technically call identification with the aggressor. Ironically, to identify with him was to identify totally with the company, for that is precisely what he called for, and she obeyed. She was a complete insider, with a complete sacrifice of her spirit, which throttled her light.

The second hole in the story was this. If she had to comply with the old man (father, professor, company), to some extent, how is it she would accept a total surrender, instead of a surrender in one (small) sector? She just assumed this was necessary in looking out at the world of school for the fall, when actually it wasn't self-evident that she had to put away her bicycle, when fall here is long and great. (See Rilke's [1938] "Autumn Day": "Lord, it is time. The summer was very big" [p. 71]). Nor did all of school, and all of social life, have to be this surrender.

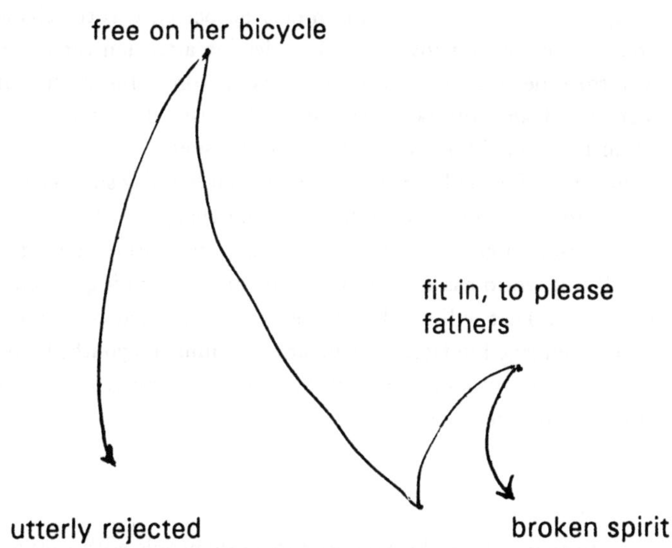

Figure 14.1. Character and the economic machinery.

She *did,* however, make further surrenders, with roommates, men, and, perhaps most importantly, in her view of her impending career in graduating from school into business. She assumed she had to surrender to corporations in New Jersey! I was, as Sullivan would say, raising her sights from being cast on the ground (Sullivan, 1956, "The Case of the Housewife Economist"; Gustafson, 1986, Chapter 6).

In summary, here is a typical dilemma of collision with the economic machinery that is deeply built into the patient's character. Reich (1933/1949) would have liked this connection of character to economy. The patient has lifted herself out of her childhood misery of being quelled by her father to identify with him as her dream of youth, which is to fit her into the economy. The selective inattention in the dream of this character merely hands her over to being utterly crushed by her success as an insider. If she goes to the shadow side in summer, finding ephemeral freedom, it merely sets her up for the fall, which will be her end. She is carried away, as an outsider, by a god like Shelly's of the West Wind, which has but a brief wildness.

There were big holes on the inside and on the outside surface, which when found, uncovered her great energy, which being somewhat wild was modulated in brief psychotherapy to a more comic, enjoyable form. I remember, in supervising the resident, her doctor, watching videotapes of her discussing interviews with the great companies of New Jersey. Instead of turning herself over to them, as to a press gang, she was quite hilarious in telling how she asked them difficult questions. It was possible to be an individual-member with spirit, while being reasonably polite!

While I am on the subject of character, I want to add that this case is typical of the brief psychotherapy I propose, in that my pointing to the two great holes in the story inevitably challenges the center of the patient's character. Built as Reich (1933/1949) proposed on an identification with a hero designed to lift the child out of helpless weakness into success in the machinery of society, it is the character that selectively attends, outside and inside. If the selective attention carries the child-adult to success, then the holes in the attention never become problematic. If they do lead to disaster, and I am able point this out, then the character is shaken and threatens to drop the adult back to the child's helplessness.

While I agree with Reich (1933/1949) and his modern-day successor, Davanloo (1986), that character is the great limitation to a big change, I do not agree that it needs to be browbeaten about its array of defenses, its posture, and its constant attitude. After all, the world has already shaken its grip by striking it from the side, where it had no sight. That will do. I just need to take up that collision, not force another one. We are engaged in facing the dream of a child and youth, hardened into the armor of character, now shaken and coming apart. The stakes are very high, and require a revision of the ancient dream.

Society

To have company in this world, you need to locate people with similar interests or pursuits. It is parallel play that is possible, enjoying each others' qualities as you chase the rabbit, or the buck, or the status, and so forth. These are hunting or increase packs. You get company by being a member in good standing. (See Chapter 4, "Male Dilemmas" for a full discussion of increase packs. Women nowadays are often full, if slighted, participants in these proceedings, or they have a comparable and traditional pack of mothers, householders, gatherers, or the like. In Bion's terms, the increase pack operates on a basic fight–flight assumption, the mother pack on a basic dependency assumption. In other words, the pack behavior is instinctual and strictly governed by innate releasing mechanisms.(See Gustafson, 1995, Chapter 18, for further discussions.))

This would appear to be perfectly obvious, but I can tell you it is certainly not obvious to my patients. I have many who complain of no society when they have no interests or pursuits, as if company would suddenly turn up for somebody who is no fun at all. I have many who have interests and pursuits but are easily crushed, and so they have to enjoy themselves in secret while they complain to me of loneliness. Finally, I have many patients who find people to fall in with for fun, but then find that they are not allowed to change the subject to anything else! This amazes and aggrieves them, as if something unusual is happening. Then, they are either mad, or hurt, or vaguely thinking that something is wrong with them.

Many fail to meet their quotas in the increase packs of work and then hope to have it made up by society. They find that society is also thinly connected (Gustafson and Cooper, 1990) by another set of increase packs, that of socializing. Churches, dinner parties, PTAs, Masons, political causes, softball teams, and the like turn out to have same structure. They have a ritual or game you can fall in with, and then they disperse. The ritual or game is about increasing something, like money or prestige or runs.

In the opening pages of *War and Peace,* Tolstoy (1869/1966) describes a typical socializing event, a soiree of Anna Pavlovna Scherer, which he compares to a spinning mill:

> As the foreman of a spinning mill, when he has set the hands to work, goes round and notices here a spindle that has stopped or there one that creaks or makes more noise than it should, and hastens to check the machine or set it in proper motion, so Anna Pavlovna moved about her drawing room, approaching now a silent, now a too-noisy group, and by a word or slight rearrangement kept the conversational machine in steady, proper, and regular motion. (p. 10)

Tolstoy makes it entirely clear that his machinery is for allocating prestige. Prestige, in turn, is symbolic capital (Bourdieu, 1977) that can be turned into literal capital, because the connections made in the drawing room can be drawn upon for getting appointments in the ministries and in the army, and for arranging marriages.

Of course, brilliant success in the army and brilliant success in society do not necessarily do much for a person's soul. Prince Andrew responds to Scherer's soiree with bitterness and gloom, because he has been through it all thousands of times, and it is ever the same show. Even if he is doubly brilliant outside, he is filled inside with darkness. Those who take it seriously, like Anna and Prince Vasili, come across as weary, empty puppets, fabricating enthusiasm. Only the young get much out of it, projecting their own vitality and playfulness onto the dead machinery.

It is terrible for those who fail doubly, like Anna Mikhaylovna, a faded princess on the margin who can arrange no appointments for her son, Boris. She is, thus, doubly alienated from the economy and from the society. She would be a typical patient coming to our clinic.

A Case of Alienation in a Graduate Student of English

A young female graduate student came in for depression, but she was also quite anxious, like nearly every patient who comes for a first visit. She had been all right until she took a prelim exam that she failed badly and unexpectedly. She was going to take it again, but she found herself unable to do the reading. This made her anxious, and she slept poorly. She had no one to talk to about this, as she felt her peers would not want to hear it, having their own struggles. As for faculty, she just feared them. She was doubly alienated, failing her increase toward her thesis, and failing to have any company in her sorrow and dread.

I knew she was very frightened, for she startled and drew back when the resident brought her around the corner and ran into me. I also knew she was brimming with grief and yet unable to get relief, because the resident would take her right up to it, and yet she wouldn't let go with her tears.

Many graduate students in the humanities have schizoid personalities, which means they arrange security by being half in and half out of relationships. In work they use their chief talent, their minds, leaving their hearts out of their dry topics. Thus, in work and in society, their characters dispose them to be lonely, while they dread full engagement even more. Now, if I test engagement, I can find out if they feel relieved by being understood, or if they feel worse and get demanding. The first response is what Balint called a "benign regression" and the second a "malignant regression." The first group do well in psychotherapy, and the second group get worse and worse the more they are helped.

I needed to see if she could get any comfort from being understood, and so, during my turn to interview, I simply commented that she was very upset. Her eyes moistened, but she braced herself with both arms as if beyond reach in a fortress. Two arms horizontally encasing the chest signal a very strong reluctance to open up, and must be addressed if feelings are to flow. (A single arm diagonally across the chest, usually the right arm reaching up to the left shoulder, is a variation. It has a double defensive duty, to shield the heart and to be positioned for striking out backhandedly at an intruder.) She told me she ought not to be upset, because others in her peer group did not seem to be upset. I replied that they only looked like they were coping, but we were taking care of all fifty of them, secretly and individually. She smiled at this, and eased the tension in her arms. I added that while she ought not to be upset, she actually was. She let down her tears.

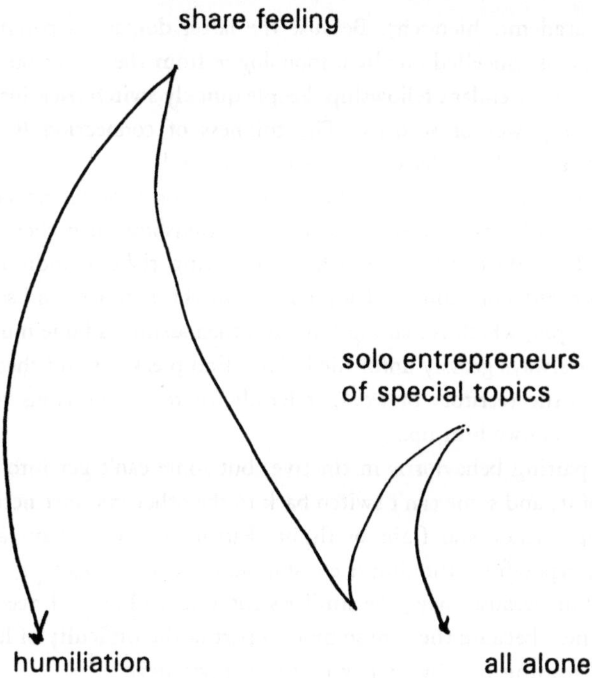

Figure 14.2. Double alienation.

I discovered, by inquiry, that she had had closer friends earlier in graduate school. At the beginning, when they arrived from various points of the compass, they had openly been a comfort to each other, but an insidious distance had set in as each went the way of his or her own specialty. Each became a kind of solo entrepreneur, quite like the mentors higher up in the hierarchical machinery—the professors. The society of the English Department turned out to be quite like Anna Scherer's soiree, with everybody trying to look as brilliant as they could while hiding their distress. Doubly alienated, from its economy and society, she needed us.

Love

To have individual and close relationships, you need to find someone with whom you can be indiscreet and say what is not allowed in society. Naturally, there are all degrees of indiscretion. There may always be topics that exceed the degree or range worked out between friends.

The tricky part about friendship is knowing its mutual domain, and where it crosses over into being expressive for one friend and injurious and, thus, perverse, for another friend. This can be hard to reckon, because a fine conversation that began in a seminar of mutual interest may pass rapidly into another domain, say, career-making in an academic hierarchy. Because the latter domain is paramount to one speaker, the first is cancelled out by a monologue from the career builder that fits him nicely into his ascendant fellowship. People quickly switch back into the conversational lanes of power or security. The thinness of connection (Gustafson and Cooper, 1990) can be bewildering if it is not expected.

This is not as obvious as the mechanics of work and society, and so my patients have even more difficulty reckoning personal relationships than they do work and societal ones. They do not know much about taking risks of indiscretion and so nothing is ventured nor gained. They engage in the simplest indiscretion of all between two people, which is making love, and then assume a huge mutual interest, which is almost always grossly unfulfilled. They find pleasures and then are shocked by returning to the territory of work or family, or to the previous society of the friend, which swallows him up.

In brief, pairing behavior is instinctive, but some can't get into it, and some can't get out of it, and some can't switch back to the other two instinctive territorial patterns of dependency and fight or flight. Pairing is apt to have a very erratic history. I am purposefully running friendship and sexuality together, not because I equate them, but because they pose similar structural problems. I need to bring up these subjects here because they are so much a part of the difficulty of looking out at the world and reading in it what is going to happen next.

Jung's Dilemma and Romance

There is an interesting relationship between a society of increase packs and romance that was certainly well known to Shakespeare and expressed in his *Romeo and Juliet*. The more barren the society in its narrow-minded increase packs, the greater the pressure that builds for pairing to provide bliss. Romeo and Juliet get outside the perpetual quarrels of the Montagues and the Capulets. Of course, their bliss is transient, crushed by the cruel forces of the envious packs.

This is precisely what Jung was pointing to when he suggests that freeing from society it apt to get you swept away by gods, in this instance, gods of love. This is utterly routine with eighteen-year-olds, and so we have four billion people on the earth created by their unions. We also have a divorce rate of 50 percent, which shows how such unions may be fertile for keeping the race going, but miserable for a sustaining love. And from what I can read between the lines in my city, the 50 percent who stay married may be more like Anna Scherer and Prince Vasili, more conventional than substantial.

A Case of Three Husbands

This woman has lived through two of the disasters of marriage and is contemplating a third. She met her first husband in law school, and they had a great trip to

Europe together. All was well until they settled in his hometown so he could join his father's big law practice. She came along and got a job running a social service agency.

As soon as they got to town, her husband got anxiously involved in proving himself as the suspect son of the senior partner. When he was home, he watched television. When she complained of having disappeared from his horizon, he withdrew further into the television. When she complained of the dreadful holidays at his parents', surrounded by the anxious hierarchy of the law firm, he withdrew even more and complained to his father of her disloyalty. Here was a man who was good company in Europe, and yet his shadow was withdrawal when the going got difficult. Of course, he didn't want marital help, either. She left him.

Her second husband was more passionate, and angrily detached from his family. He was full of deep interests to share. It went well, like all the other archetypal pairs of history who depart society. As soon as she began to ask for his help, he turned on her with equal and now negative passion and crushed her as an excessively dependent lady. It was relevant that, with great bitterness, he had taken care of his five younger brothers and sisters. She got his wrath, when she appeared like them, as needful. He didn't want marital help, either. She left him.

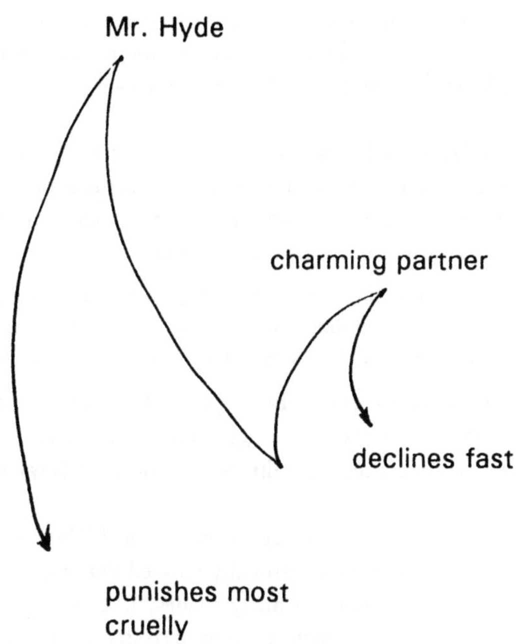

Figure 14.3. Reading men.

Now she contemplates a third husband. This Lochinvar is gentle toward her needfulness, unlike the second husband, and is not a man to run away from feelings. She is in love again, hoping to surpass her two previous misadventures. I say to her that I am glad Lochinvar has come out of the West, but I myself have no way of reading the shadow of his character. It is too soon to tell, for she is now getting his best foot forward, and they have not yet had a single collision of their interests. Only when they do collide will she see his shadow. The first husband ran from conflict, the second was merciless, and the prospective third? For the sake of symmetry, perhaps he would surrender and get depressed. Then she would have a complete education in the three presenting characters of mankind, and their three shadows. I told her that because of her history I could not trust her conscious standpoint on men, and could only wait for her unconscious to balance it with dreams. And she herself would not get this reading if she jumped in in haste, as was her wont. Perhaps she had had enough dire experience with mankind to take the time to estimate his character in shadow. I concluded that she is bound to fail a third time if her third husband lacks the character to cope with differences equably. The first marriage lasted nine years, and took three years of psychotherapy to face its impossibility; the second, one year and took a much briefer reckoning.

COVER-UP AND AMAZEMENT

I will return to the prospect of utilizing dreams as a second unconscious eye to assist the conscious eye to see around its selective inattention to the hierarchy of society in the domains of work, society, and love. Together, the two eyes provide a full view of the social world.

Before I conclude, I need to say something about the cover-up that obscures much of the universe of human hierarchy and the amazement of the perceiver who is taken in by the outer show. Orwell (1946) has the most memorable picture for me of the deception that is routine with respect to power:

> The great enemy of clear language is insincerity. When there is a gap between one's real and one's declared aims, one turns as it were instinctively to long words and exhausted idioms, like a cuttlefish squirting out ink. (p. 167)

Nouns are best for hiding under. Every period has its formulae. "Concern" is a favorite here in Madison. It is cheaply bought and used, especially by professionals. Even car salesmen are concerned to help us get the best buys without pressure. Imagine that!

How are our patients to see through these covers? They won't if they aren't looking, and they won't if they are continually amazed that the cover has little to do with the book. Amazement comes in many shades, like surprise, frustration, perplexity, upset, and shock. If amazement is allowed to stand, the patient is sure to get hit by the same thing again unawares. It is the tone of amazement that is the telltale sign of selective inattention. It means there is a big hole in the patient's outward view. This is Sullivan's (1956, Chapter 3; Gustafson, 1986, Chapter 6) greatest discovery, and hardly a therapist knows anything about it, a huge weakness in the psychotherapy establishment. Every patient mentioned in this chapter was amazed, and would continue to be hurt if I had not taken up his amazement. It is guaranteed.

The signs are there, alongside the pretence. Listen to Tolstoy's (1875) description of a famous, concerned attorney for divorces:

> He was as spruce as a bridegroom, from his white necktie and double watch-chain to his patent leather boots. . . . But hardly had he settled down when a moth flew across the table. The lawyer, with a rapidity one could not have expected of him, separated his hands, caught the moth, and resumed his former position. (p. 333)

We do not miss the detail—Tolstoy repeats the snagging of the moth three times! It is no accident in such a predator so full of concern.

THE EYE OF THE UNCONSCIOUS

Our patients are going to miss the snatching of the moth, even if it occurs three hundred times, because they want to believe in the concern of their attorney, their beloved, or their department. Such faith will miss everything but what it wants to find.

I always tell these souls that the conscious standpoint is hopelessly inadequate unless compensated by the unconscious, from dreams. Let me close with two simple examples.

A Case of Three Husbands, Revisited

My patient, after two divorces and looking toward a third marriage, did some dating. She was looking for concern in a man that would take care of her well. She met a new man, and dreamt thus:

> We are going out and he needs to stop at a Stop and Go store. I pull into the shadows, watching, and he comes out. There is a man leaning against his car, waiting for him. He takes out a knife and slits him from throat to anus and takes out his heart and eats it.

She had dimly felt he was a lonely, hungry man, but little did she imagine just how hungry he was going to become. If the dream was exaggerated it made its point, and she realized her conscious standpoint about him was going to underestimate his needfulness. She decided to turn elsewhere.

A Case of Idealism in a Scientist, Corrected

Dreams can focus on the god that would possess us, and they can also look outward to the world we mis-estimate to picture its requirements. Jung said little about the latter, but it is a great resource for our patients. This young man was going to a scientific meeting in San Francisco with a young colleague, hoping to show off their exciting discovery. He dreamt thus:

> I am riding with my friend in a curious box in San Francisco. It fits into a kind of railroad, like those boxes that fit on freight cars. The two of us, sitting in the box, are being transported, without any control from us, down a track full of similar boxes, which is crossed at many angles by other tracks, full of similar boxes. I wake up in a panic, feeling we have no control at all, and might be smashed at any moment.

His unconscious gave him, if exaggerated, a pretty good picture of a scientific meeting to correct his conscious optimism. They would be two, among countless, and their box (discovery) might be received in any which way by the powers that be in their field. This dream allowed us to discuss, as it were, how they proposed to score in terms of how scoring is reckoned in their field. This settled him down, for now he is attuned to his increase pack, rather than going out of control, full of enthusiasm for his findings.

Chapter 15

Ten Follow-up Evaluations and the Science of Brief Psychotherapy

The poetry of science may be very fine in its creation of hypotheses, but it is still necessary to subject them to rigorous tests (Gustafson, 1986, Chapter 17; Maturana and Varela, 1980; Popper, 1934). After all, Einstein's theory of relativity is a marvelous construction, but it could have been wrong. The Michaelson–Morley experiments were thus of great importance.

Conversely, science depends upon the art for the creation of hypotheses that are more than trivial. Popper (1934) was very interested in Adler's ideas about the baleful influence of the inferiority complex, until he discovered that Adler found the same influence in every case. Adler's one idea is a typical verbal formula that puts everything else into shadow, where it lacks form, amorphous as Sullivan [1956, Chapter 12] describes. There is a reductive tendency in the science of psychotherapy in which hypotheses are kept simple enough to study, but the study no longer concerns the actual complexity of psychotherapy. A pale and watered down in vitro study substitutes for the actual study of in vivo psychotherapy.

The art of psychotherapy is a complex activity, like any other art. The word *art* comes from the Latin *ars,* which means to fit together, as in the word *artus,* which means a joint. For me, art has to utilize the full faculties to do justice to the difficulties of the life of a patient. A study that is reduced to the cognitive faculty, the behavioral, the emotional-psychodynamic, or the willful-strategic is pale indeed. It may show that you can do something with limited means, and that is worth knowing. But it tells us little about the full force of a drama that has all of its faculties, and has not been dismembered.

Much progress in Western science has been possible because of the reductive approaches. They boil complexity down in a test tube, distilling ingredients, like getting alcohol out of grain. It's true that alcohol is a powerful drug, but it is not the same as the living field of grain. The field of grain has a complex ecology, which is grasped by the reverse of reductive science (Allen and Starr, 1982). As Allen and Starr argue, reductive science has been helpful in systems that are very small-number simple systems and very large-number simple systems:

> The former group is treated appropriately by differential equations (e.g., planets) and in the latter case statistical approaches to the entities replace exact values with averages (e.g., gas laws). . . . Nevertheless, as the interrelationship between parts (entities or averages) increases in complexity, then both calculus and statistics quickly reach the limits of their analytic power. (p. xi)

A different kind of science concerns the so-called middle-number systems:

> These are cases where there are too few parts to average their behavior reliably and too many parts to manage each separately with its own equation. . . . A statistical treatment of a system *whose parts are importantly heterogeneous* gives fuzzy results—not worthless but certainly more vague than would be fully satisfactory. . . . massive reductionist simulations seem to have offered all the insightful summary they can. (pp. xi–xii; my italics)

Allen and Starr's summary of large-number approaches and small-number approaches to middle-number systems in biology is pretty close to a summary of the results of psychotherapy research, namely, vague and reductive. What they propose instead for the field of ecology are models that can grasp the complex interaction of different levels of organization.

Bateson wrote:

> Every evolutionary step is an addition of information to an already existing system. Because this is so, the combinations, harmonies and discords between successive pieces and layers of information will present many problems of survival and determine many directions of change. . . . But, as of 1978, there is no conventional method of describing this tangle. (Bateson, 1979, quoted in Gustafson, 1986, p. 349)

Notice the musical metaphor, which is apt, because music can create such structures that oscillate between different levels of organization.

For example, in our field of psychotherapy, the strength of motive, or what is called motivation, is one level of organization, and the availability of work in a viable economy is another level of organization. A complex problem concerns the interaction of motive in a particular person to work, and the ecology of working possibilities. Allen and Starr (1982) note well that the pattern of such interaction will remain opaque unless we model using hierarchies:

> By hierarchy is understood a system of behavioral interconnections wherein the higher levels constrain and control the lower levels to various degrees depending upon the time constraints of the behavior. . . . Since bulkier structures in biology generally behave more slowly, not only do slow entities constrain fast, but also large entities constrain small. (p. xiv)

Thus, it seems very important to me that something like the outer world of the economy, or the outer world of social grouping—those bulky selecting structures for the availability of work and love—be brought into focus in order to understand their constraining of individual performances, which we measure as the outcome of psychotherapy. The individual who has the right orientation, and the right degree of motive power, still has to break through these large constraining forces to become successful in work and love, the two great desiderata of the success of psychotherapy ever since Freud proclaimed them so. I think the science of psychotherapy has to be hierarchical to bring into focus these differential levels of organization so germane to success or tragedy.

A VERY BRIEF HISTORY OF THE SCIENCE OF PSYCHOTHERAPY RESEARCH IN COMPLEX TERMS

There has been some modest success in modeling and measuring psychotherapy as a complex project with a hierarchical structure "whose parts are importantly heterogenous" (Allen and Starr, 1982, p. xii), as opposed to the usual procedure of flattening it out into a sheet of factors and grouping the input factors versus the output factors in statistical terms. I will briefly review the work of Malan, Luborsky *et al.*, and Gustafson.

Malan's Contribution

For me, Malan's chief contribution is his distinction between symptomatic and *dynamic change* (Malan, 1963, 1976a,b). Symptomatic change is the flat concept of a list of symptoms (such as the SCL-90) which either shift statistically, or not, over time. Dynamic change is a hierarchical concept that collects a set of symptoms as a maladaptive response to a defined set of situations that the patient falters over.

Barry Palmer (personal communication) describes the distinction between flat statistics and hierarchical clarity of interaction as follows:

> But in my own view it was the poet and anthropologist Ruth Benedict who came closest to the elusive quest, only five days before her death. She had studied five American Indian tribes. Three suicidal, disintegrating, miserable, two healthy, high-spirited, and well functioning. Over fifty "independent variables" thought to "cause" these differences had failed entirely to predict the outcomes. Benedict moved to a different paradigm. What mattered, she decided, was not the presence of a particular variable, say, self-interest or altruism, but the *synergy between the two*. Societies were happy when the two values had been reconciled, miserable when each fought the other. Her unpublished papers were found by Abraham Maslow, who made synergy the cornerstone of his theories. The individual must be reconciled to social concerns, he taught;

> altruism and egoism must coevolve. Which brings us back to our welfare system and the need for a logic that transcends the warring "rationalities . . . synergy of self-interest/altruism."

The test of dynamic change is to look at new instances of the difficult set or class of situations to see if the patient finds new and adaptive responses, which, in turn, will be reflected in the reduction of symptoms. For example, a patient may get highly symptomatic when he is faced with aggressive confrontations. A reduction in symptoms per se or a significant statistical change in symptoms may actually mean nothing about change in psychotherapy. It looks good, but the patient may merely be more successfully running away from confrontations, and be weaker! Thus, the cowardly lion in *The Wizard of Oz* could get psychotherapy after which he hides out even more, like a mouse in a hole. He is free of fear, but he actually has less confidence every day. The usual procedure of assessing symptomatic change will be fooled in this case where the cowardly lion has changed into a cowardly mouse. An assessment of dynamic change will ask if the lion has faced any new hazards on the yellow brick road and if he is still turning tail and quaking, or giving battle and feeling more brave. The hierarchical concept of dynamic change *poses a hierarchy of situations,* in which some are more significant than others, namely, the class of situations that test the weak capacity of the patient in question.

For me, Malan's other big idea is his decision to privilege *motivation* and *focus* as the two classes of input that are significant to the output of dynamic change. Again, he is using hierarchical concepts, which propose that some activities in psychotherapy are more significant than others. For Malan, motivation is the availability of motive to work in psychotherapy on what the patient is asked to do for his part in the work: namely, bring up his problems, feel things deeply, think about the patterns interpreted to him, and risk new experiments in behavior. In other words, motivation is motive in terms of will, feeling, cognition, and behavior. It is the patient's part, for which he has readiness or not, and to varying degrees it can be quantified. Focus for Malan is the therapist's contribution to deciding what is worth looking at and what is to be brushed aside as relatively irrelevant. For Malan, focus is a very cognitive idea for summarizing the therapist's contribution, which Malan imagined in terms of the interpretations that are recommended by psychoanalysts.

With these hierarchical constructs, Milan (1976a, 1976b) made some surprising discoveries. He found that chronic neurotics could make dynamic changes in brief psychotherapy if motivation and focus were high. He found that patients with high motivation (star cases) did very well even in disorderly group therapy (Malan *et al.*, 1976) and in long-term psychotherapy (Malan, 1976a, 1976b). Even in single sessions of intake evaluation, when the patient could not be accepted for treatment, these highly motivated patients utilized well-focused remarks from the intake team to go ahead on their own to make significant dynamic changes (Malan *et al.*, 1975). With five- to ten-year follow-ups, these star cases could number as many as a quarter of the cases, and they could remember very well what was said to them that made such a big difference. Evidently, orientation that sorts out what is going to make the patient worse from what is going to make him better goes a very long way if the patient is motivated to work on improving himself.

Luborsky et al.

Luborsky et al. (1988) continue Malan's project in terms of dynamic change (Health-Sickness Rating Scale) and focus (Core-Conflictual Relationship Theme) and add attention to the helping alliance as a felt partnership between patient and doctor. In effect, they are broadening the focus of the therapeutics from a cognitive orientation about what is wrong to a feeling orientation of connecting to the patient. This is obviously a strong point, and it shows in their results, because a patient is unlikely to listen to the most cogent of interpretations if he dislikes or distrusts the therapist, and, further, he is likely to go forward better if he has been found and comforted in emotional as well as cognitive terms. *It helps very much to have an ally, as well as a good map.* Luborsky *et al.* demonstrate that both are critical to outcome on long-term follow-up.

There are many other sound and interesting confirmations of the validity of this pair of values in psychotherapy—the ally and the map. For example, Strupp and his colleagues found that college professors could do better than professional therapists when they allied themselves warmly with their student patients (see Strupp and Binder [1984] for a summary and further references). Korsch and Negrete (1972) found that mothers in a pediatric emergency room showed huge differences in cooperation with the doctors' orders for their child when they were reached in terms of their fear and guilt. Werner's (1989) study of nearly seven hundred children from prenatal exams to their thirties showed spectacular differences in outcome for children from extremely disastrous homes. The difference was motivation to get out of the home catastrophe and find some relative, neighbor, teacher, or coach to be an ally. Those who sat in the home wilted, while those determined to get out flowered, over thirty years. Werner felt it was a matter of constitution to some degree. Some children seemed hardier and determined from the word go.

Gustafson

In my first book (Gustafson, 1986), I accepted the validity of Malan's findings concerning motivation and focus leading to dynamic change. My criticism was that this analysis left out the world, especially the systemic world of possibilities in the family and in the hierarchy of the economy. While it was well and good to say that a patient with a great deal of motive power who is met by a therapist with a clear focus on what is wrong with the investment of that motive power is going to have a better chance of getting somewhere, this still leaves out the world in which there are sometimes more and sometimes less opportunities for investment. This is partic-

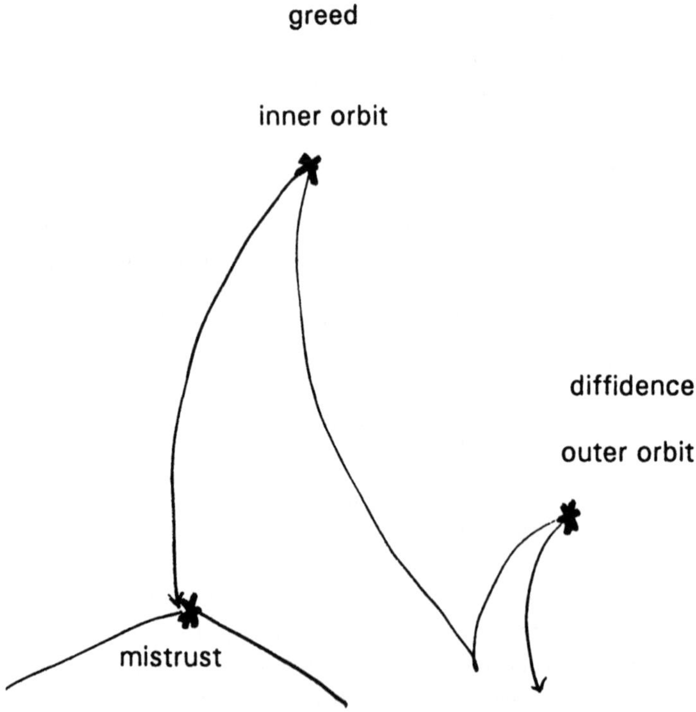

Figure 15.1. Strange attractors (3).

ularly clear nowadays, when we are so aware that families can be extremely cruel, as can hierarchies of business, academia, government, and so forth. A young person who is highly motivated and clearly focused may do very badly in the long run, when his family cannot get behind him through a long series of disappointments that are typical nowadays in finding a place in the world, or when he is coming out of a sector of the social and economic world in which everybody fails for lack of viable work (such as from the ghetto or reservation). Thus, I argued for attention to systemic change, and gave such attention (in addition to symptomatic and dynamic change) for seventeen cases, mostly in brief psychotherapy. Compared to Malan and Luborsky, with their teams of researchers and blind assessments, my studies were not terribly rigorous. I simply gave attention myself to following up seventeen cases with some attention to the power of the world.

Then I reviewed Luborsky et al. (Gustafson, 1989) and outlined some crucial weaknesses, which I address in the ten follow-up interviews that follow in this chapter. First, I argued that interpretation of core conflicts may be a good idea, but like all good ideas, it is about half right. There are extremely vigorous forces that resist the reasonableness of good ideas. I called them mistrust, greed, and diffidence. I noted that Balint (1952) had preceded me in this criticism, with his remarks concerning his own practice. Mistrust, or the paranoid position, held many in place. Greed, or the depressive position, held many in place. Diffidence was my idea, as a kind of capitulation to conformity to get a place.

Now, I would say that mistrust and greed keep patients in an inner orbit that refuses to be budged by the constraints of the outer world. Diffidence locks patients in an outer orbit, where they lose themselves. Thus, the rule is for the inner orbit and the outer orbit to become disconnected. The patient lives around either the inner or the outer as a kind of strange attractor. Thus, a patient may be diffident in her work, fearing to claim anything, while she is a raging lioness at home claiming all. Two strange attractors dominate her life, one diffident and one greedy. There is little connection between them, but a gulf (catastrophe) in which she switches attractors as she switches territories (work to home). Oddly, she is governed by a third attractor, mistrust, which keeps her half in and half out of the other two. As long as the two worlds are thus dissociated, there is a stasis, which is seen in the limitation of the orbit in which the patient can move. There is very little range of motion. I believe we are not apt to discover this limitation unless we are alert to looking for it.

Conversely, the patients who can move backward and forward freely between their outer orbit and their inner orbit achieve a transcendence (Jung, 1916/1971a) over the limitations of either attractor. They are not prisoners of conformity (diffidence), nor are they prisoners of their own recalcitrance (mistrust, greed). They move in this region of the equipoise, where the two attractors cancel out each other's dire opposite effects, leaving the patient to move much more freely.

Therefore, in the current study I distinguish three levels of change. Learning I is success in getting off the dire slope (orbit) of which the patient is complaining (say, confrontation in work). Learning II is success in mastering (to a greater or lesser extent) the entire class of such situations (not only work, but intimacy, family, etc.). Learning II requires some mastery of the opposite slope (of the opposite orbit). Thus, a problem in confrontation in the outer orbit will be mastered only with comfort in being helpless in the inner orbit. Learning III is transcendence in the region of the equipoise between the inner and outer orbits in terms of a complete range of emotional situations (not only confrontation, say, but also sexuality, greed, and so forth). In other words, I am distinguishing three hierarchical levels of dynamic change, compared to the single level of Malan and Luborsky.

My other criticism of Luborsky et al. was that they, like Malan, hardly mentioned the dire effects of the surrounding world in selecting what is even possible for the patients. Like Allen and Starr in their ecology, I did not want to assume that outcomes of individual creatures could be intelligently divorced from the world that gave them territory or not! So I concluded my review (Gustafson, 1989) with this summary:

> As I read over the brief characterizations of the patients in the Penn Study who succeeded versus those who failed, I thought it could be put most simply in ecological terms: The successful patients found they had something to give to

> the world and found a way to arrange a better give and take for themselves. The unsuccessful patients seemed to feel empty, cheated and fearful, and so long as they were lost in such patterns, it is little wonder that they did not connect well with the worlds that might be open to them. (p. 52)

Therefore, I have enlarged my conception of therapeutic beyond Malan and Luborsky, including their concepts of motivation and focus, adding my concept of available territory. Thus, I look for whether patients have sufficient motive, whether they become well oriented, and whether they have places to land (I am grouping the helpful alliance noted by Luborsky et al. under motive power)! I hypothesize that they need force to go forward with an ally, an accurate orientation to the topography of their dilemma (as opposed to having major gaps of cloudiness or selective inattention), and available landings: *ally, map, and places*.

TEN FOLLOW-UP STUDIES

I make no claim that these ten studies are proof for my methods of brief psychotherapy. These studies lack the rigor that can only be supplied by large teams of researchers, where the therapists have no part in studying the outcome of their own patients (in which they have to be very biased), and where the researchers who set up the criteria for change are completely separate from the researchers who evaluate the patients according to the advance criteria.

Also, these studies are mostly of cases conducted by trainees with a very slight understanding of what I recommend in this book or do on a daily basis in my office. There is no rigorous test of my methods; in fact, there is hardly a test of my methods at all. Nevertheless, I think the reader will find the studies very interesting in terms of the possibilities opened up for the rigorous study of complex hierarchical work in psychotherapy. These studies give me a chance to show what I believe is powerful in the drama of our work. Also, they show the drama of dilemmas over time. They could be said to be studies more of the passage of time than of the effects of psychotherapy.

Yet some large shifts in orientation seem to occur even in single sessions with highly motivated patients who have available territory to move into in a new way. I, therefore, divide the cases into three groups. The first group of four shows these drastic shifts in orientation in highly motivated patients with available territory. The second group of two shows some of the recalcitrance that will occur when the motivation is compromised by the difficult topography of the patient's far/near (basic fault) dilemma. The third group of four illustrates the difference that availability of territory versus lack of availability of territory makes to success or tragedy. Thus, I emphasize orientation, motivation, and territory, in that order, as the limiting powers. Orientation, motive power, and territory fold in all the compartments of the

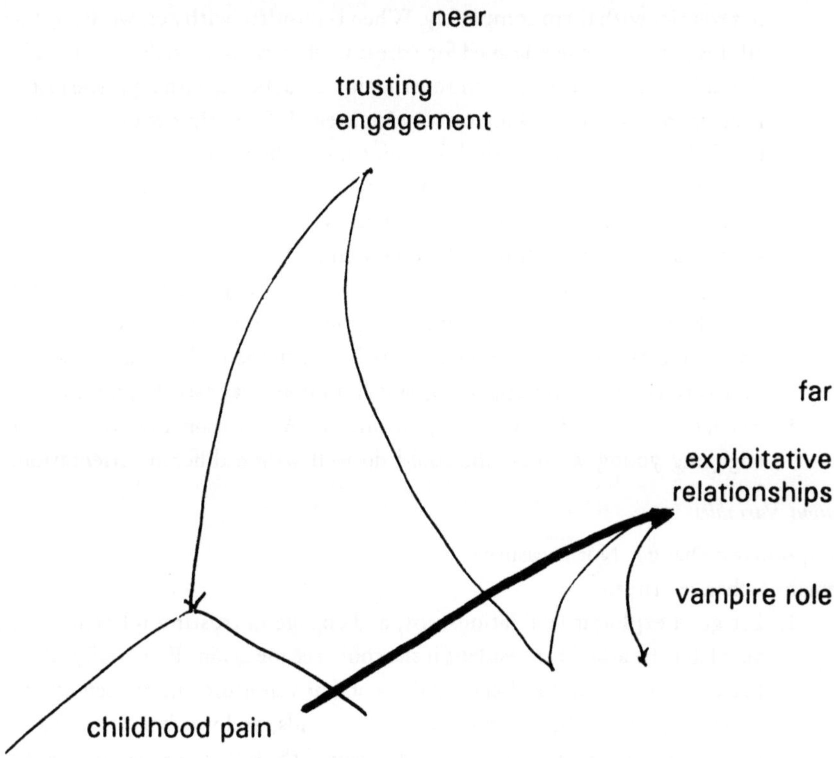

Figure 15.2. Vampire space.

psyche deemed powerful: orientation is cognitive and perceptive; motive power is affective and willful; territory is contextual and systemic.

Ally, Map, and Places

Case 1. A Vampire

Patient's age: 21. Sex: Female. Marital status: Single. Occupation: Student. Sessions: 10 by resident, 1 by myself in videotaped consultation. Psychopharmacology: None
Length of follow-up: 1 year after consultation. Setting of follow-up: Videotaped interview in Brief Therapy Clinic.

Input Variables

1. Orientation (focus): The patient was brought for consultation by the resident from a psychotherapy that was focused upon her great disappointments with her family from early childhood, and her debate with herself whether

to sever ties with them completely. When I consulted with her, we did get into all this pain, but when I asked for a dream, when we were in deep, she told me she had the same dream over and over again, about being with a guy she just met in an apartment and waking up very frightened. From the dream work, I told her that her unconscious mind, by pointing out how much danger she was in, was compensating her conscious mind, which believed she could get away with jumping into bed with men she didn't know. She responded that these dreams always occurred after one of these new flings.

2. Topography of her dilemma (motivation and helping alliance): Very simply put, she flees the painful dependence upon her family to play a very aggressive, exploitative, vampire series of strikes upon men. She connects with me in a very trusting and appealing and humorous way (see Figure 15.2).
3. Available territory (systemic opportunities): As a reasonably attractive and engaging young woman, she could do well with a different orientation.

Output Variables

Symptomatic change: Not measured

Dynamic change criteria

1. Let go of exploitative relationships, and engage in trusting relationships: A year later she asked her resident if she could see me again. Essentially, she had been very struck by our dream analysis of that single dream, had left off much of her exploits in the realm of one-night stands, and was beginning to see a man she might trust. In this second dream of the follow-up, we reached back to the innocent girl before the disaster in her family, and now I had to warn her of being overly trusting and swinging too far back. Her unconscious showed that her delight in her trusting girl-self could be too open.
2. More engagement/trust in other domains: Indeed, a year later she also had a new girlfriend who knew her better than anybody ever had.
3. (Transcendence): She obviously has a great deal of potential for using dreams, being a quick learner in two hours, but it is very early in her maturation, long held up by an interruption that was the tragedy of her childhood happiness.

DISCUSSION: Here is a lovely example of Malan's kind, of star cases jumping ahead with single sessions, which were right on the mark in terms of orienting the patient to what is dangerous for them. Certainly, the ongoing work with the resident created a holding environment in which she could practice being engaged, while the single consultation pointed exactly to her conscious mind having selective inattention for the great danger in her exploits.

Case 2. The Mythical Dimensions of J. Crew

Patient's age: 25. Sex: Female. Marital status: Single. Occupation: Student. Sessions: 20 by resident, 1 consultation by myself. Psychopharmacology: None

Length of follow-up: 1 year after consultation. Setting of follow-up: Videotaped interview in Brief Therapy Clinic.

Input Variables

1. Orientation (focus): See Chapter 3 for narrative. Essentially, I took the dream of the smiling mask of her dead friend with a crack down the middle to mean her fear of getting through her own mask (persona) to intense feeling.
2. Topography of her dilemma (motivation and helping alliance): See Figure 3.1. Consultation showed great readiness to get out of her mask and into her shadow with great feeling.
3. Available territory (systemic opportunities): She is reasonably placed as an attractive young woman with academic talent to step out of the role of pleasant object.

Output Variables

Symptomatic change: Not measured
Dynamic change criteria

1. Essentially, to step out of being a pleasing object, with low self-regard, dependent upon applause: What she discovered in the dream analysis of being chased by bears was her fear of primitive power in others and in herself. She could engage it in the dream, but I have no data on how much she could own it and modulate it to keep from scaring others away.
2. More empowerment in other domains: She was thinking about it in terms of choice of career, but had made no commitments.
3. (Transcendence): Again, just beginning to connect to the powers of the shadow world, and detach the pulls to the right.

DISCUSSION: Very similar to Case 1, showing the power of single-dream analysis to penetrate being locked into a persona, to start some assimilation of the unconscious power.

Case 3. The French Bullet Train

Patient's age: 32. Sex: Male. Marital status: Married. Occupation: Businessman. Sessions: 13 in 4 months by myself, privately. Psychopharmacology: None Length of follow-up: 4 years. Setting of follow-up: Videotaped interview in Brief Therapy Clinic with criteria for dynamic change defined in advance.

Input Variables

1. Orientation (focus): See Chapter 8 for narrative. Essentially, I pointed toward his selective inattention (amazement) at the power structure requiring submission. This led to a powerful dream in session seven, of the French

bullet train, his god of a perfect system, needing to be washed off, baptized, reborn, for his spirit to be reinvigorated.
2. Topography of his dilemma (motivation and helping alliance): The patient loved to be found out, and would point to me like an approving teacher whenever I could discover his secret. He played a low-key, low-profile part, with mask, but was secretly powerful. See Figure 8.5.
3. Available territory (systemic opportunities): He had a fall-back position to a lesser but adequate job.

Output Variables

Symptomatic change: From moderate anxiety and depression on SCL-90 to virtually none.

Dynamic change criteria

1. a. Less selective inattention for cruelty: much more ready for tests at work, although nothing so grim as the test that brought him to therapy has occurred.
   b. Resilience in relation to injustice: much more humorous and detached from the world than his serious and grim self of four years ago, so there is a looseness here that can take jarring better.
2. Less selective inattention/more resilience in relation to injustice in other domains: nicely managed in-law intrusions that threw him before.
3. (Transcendence): He has pulled back from grim attachment to the world and is more playful, but has no further access to dream world, which he remembers strangely as in a dream.

DISCUSSION: Classic brief psychotherapy with powerful dynamic change as previously demonstrated by Malan. The use of the dream as the pivot of the turnaround in a deep reach into his shadow being is not classic psychoanalytic brief psychotherapy, nor is the steady focus on selective inattention to the outer world that preceded the dream dive. It is rather the burden of this book to show that such things are possible.

Case 4. Hamlet

Patient's age: 20. Sex: Male. Marital status: Single. Occupation: Student. Sessions: Estimated 52 sessions by resident in 1 year and 9 months; 1 consultation by myself at outset. Psychopharmacology: None

Length of follow-up: 1 year, 9 months from initial consultation, patient still in therapy with resident. Setting of follow-up: Videotaped interview in Brief Therapy Clinic with criteria for dynamic change defined in advance.

Input Variables

1. Orientation (focus): As a sophomore when first seen, the patient was very ill at ease trying to be a business major to suit his mother. He was playing the

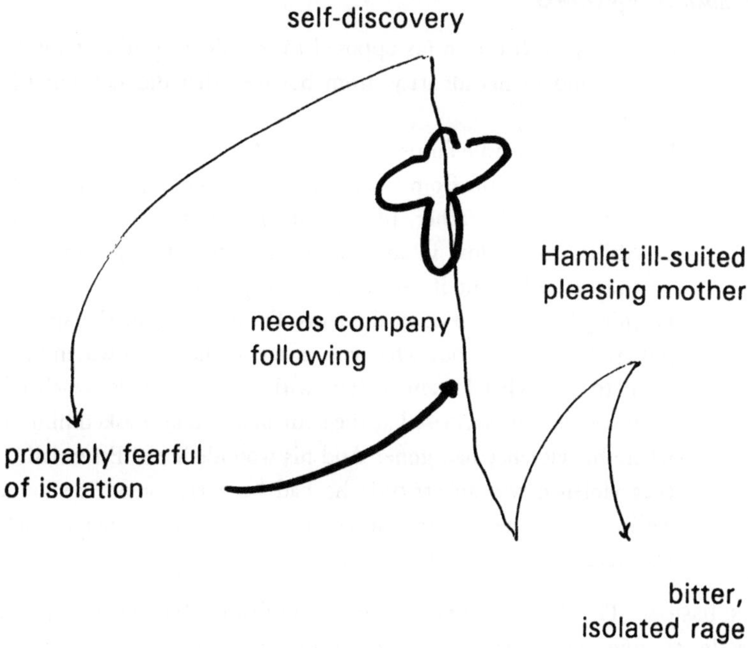

Figure 15.3. Elsinore.

isolate, with sunglasses and Walkman, superior and sadistic in his stories. It wasn't working, so he was depressed, frightened, wary, and a little scary to some of the women on our team. I posed the problem that being Hamlet was not going to be very promising, and discovered a very pleasant smile behind all this acting job and an interest in being a writer. The focus became his finding himself. His therapist gave him complete room to do this, and followed him along, summarizing the discoveries.

2. Topography of his dilemma (motivation and helping alliance): If he played Hamlet, he was going to be full of sadistic rage. If he went elsewhere to his discoveries, he could be very good-natured, yet he was probably needing some company to undergo this kind of journey (see Figure 15.3).
3. Available territory (systemic opportunities): He has striking talent as a writer, so this might get him some company for his journey of self-discovery outside the consulting room, especially in university writing programs. Beyond that, it could get a lot scarcer.

Output Variables

Symptomatic change: Less depressed and lonely, by far. Still anxious about romantic relationships.

Dynamic change criteria

1. a. Clarity of direction (as opposed to free-floating uncertainty): From lost to found in his identity, from business that did not suit him to writing.
   b. Ability to handle failures without helplessness or sadistic compensation: Remarkable shift from bitter rage, to challenging those who hurt him in a fair way, like father, like a best male friend, like a girlfriend.
   c. Ability to be close in an equal relationship: Just getting a taste of this and excited about it—obviously inexperienced.
2. Learning I changes in other domains: From taking his therapy as text, as he put it, to . . . find out what you mean, he has been widening the experiment to "say what I want to say" with family, friends, teachers, etc.
3. (Transcendence): Surprised at the shift in attitude, I asked him in follow-up where his violence had gone? And his woundedness? Essentially, he replied that violence was an attitude he had been trying on; he found it to be weakness, and he preferred acceptance. He no longer felt himself to be the wounded child of two years ago.

DISCUSSION: This is a remarkable maturation from alienation in a rotten Elsinore Castle, to going elsewhere to discover himself as a writer. Hamlet essentially goes back to Wittenberg to find what he likes, instead of boiling in his own juices. His attitude or orientation has pointed very differently, and, I think, very much more constructively. How sturdy or fragile is it? To what extent is it *dependent upon a university context* in which writing is *supported as a kind of home?* He hints at the absolute importance of writing, as a matter of life and death. When he can't find his meaning, he feels like pounding the typewriter, and he suggests he couldn't live without this channel of expression. The big tests will come around situations beyond the university, where less support could throw him back into a childhood series of griefs, which he thinks he is passed. He emphasizes that "the program of therapy" allowing him two years was a great help. Clearly, he needed two years to utilize it as a place for discovering his meaning, as a kind of exercise in getting from being lost to finding himself again.

Basic Faults

Case 5. The Grand Bartender

Patient's age: 42. Sex: Male. Marital status: Divorced. Occupation: Bartender. Sessions: 8 in 2 months by resident. Psychopharmacology: Valium, 5 mg.
Length of follow-up: 10 months from consultation, 8 months from termination of brief therapy. Setting of Follow-up: Videotaped interview in Brief Therapy Clinic with criteria for dynamic change defined in advance.

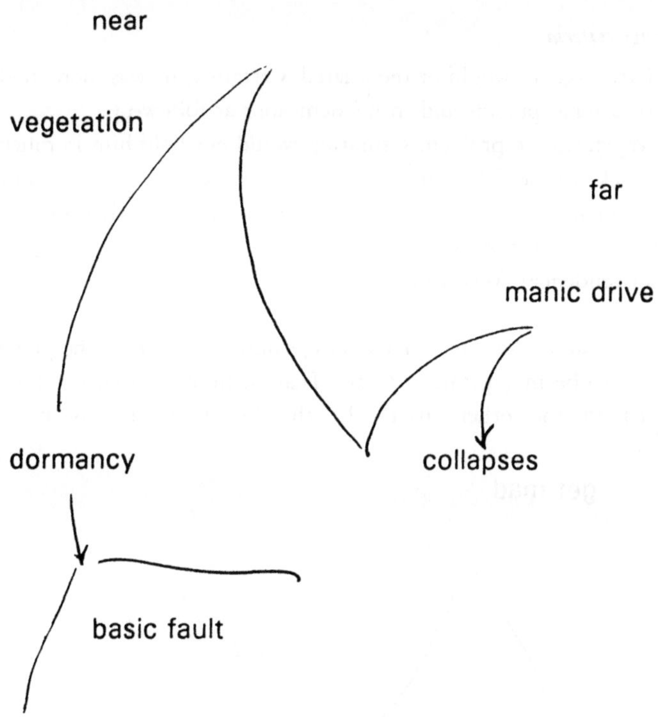

Figure 15.4. Cyclothymia.

Input Variables

1. Orientation (focus): A middle way between his manic entrepreneurial flights, and his collapses into reclusiveness.
2. Topography of his dilemma (motivation and helping alliance): Out of his sense of being a paper lion, he drove himself wildly in business, until collapse. Then, he was reclusive, vegetative, dormant (see Figure 15.4). I enjoyed his American character in its zaniness, but I am not sure he could tolerate someone close to him for long.
3. Available territory (systemic opportunities): No longer fundable for the bar business. Now he was applying for retraining in vocational rehabilitation with computers, which might be a less excessive vocation.

Output Variables

Symptomatic change: SCL-90 on follow-up shows moderate anxiety and depression. We do not have an SCL-90 for comparison, but it would be comparable to what he reported narratively.

Dynamic change criteria

1. a. Extravagance would be modulated: Certainly, he was more modest in his vocational pursuit and in his demeanor at follow-up.
   b. Vegetation in problem-saturation would not hold him in much: He was stuck here at follow-up, still on the edge of re-entry into school.
2. Extravagance and vegetation in other domains: Similarly on the edge of re-entry into an intimacy.
3. (Transcendence): Very stuck.

DISCUSSION: Classic cyclothymic character (Jacobson, 1953)—if he gets off manic drive, he tends to be in vegetative doubt. That is, he goes from one horn of his dilemma (far) to the other (near). In the follow-up it was more evident

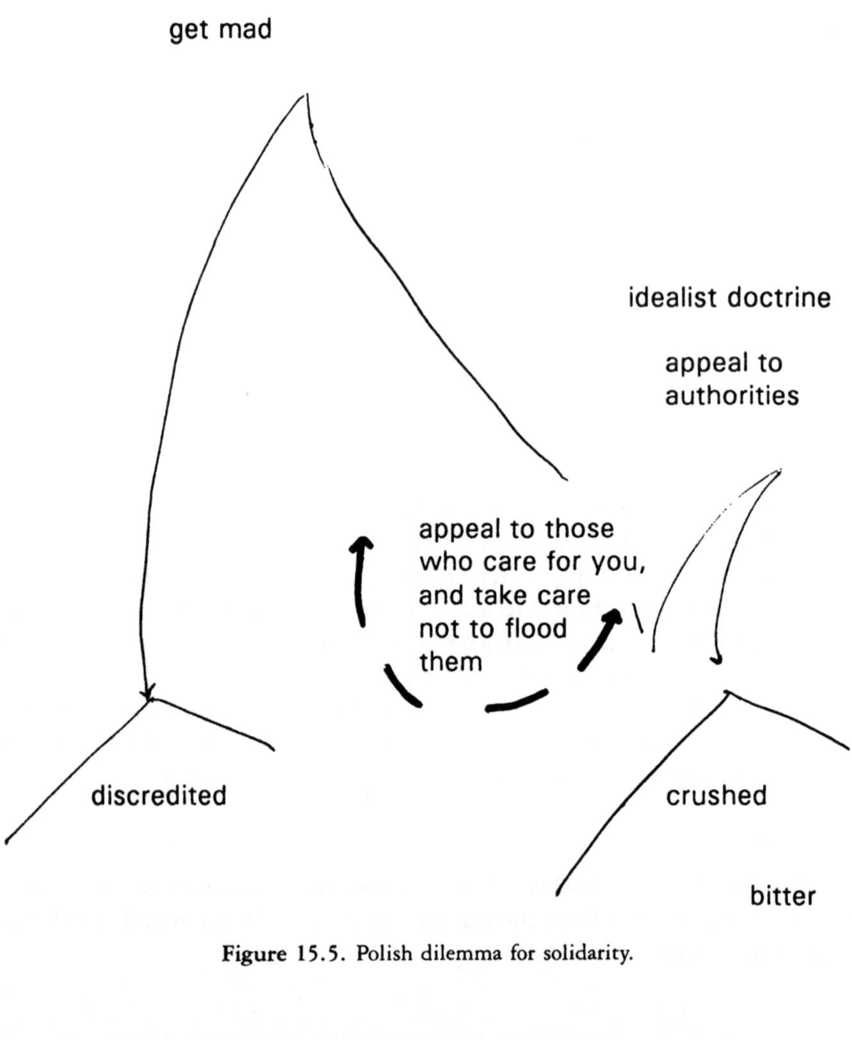

Figure 15.5. Polish dilemma for solidarity.

that he had been saddled early with the burden of his mother (basic fault of abandonment and intrusion), which thrust this dilemma upon him, of being near and swamped, or far and high.

Case 6. A Direct Young Woman (Polish Dilemma)

Patient's age: 21. Sex: Female. Marital status: Single. Occupation: Student. Sessions: Estimated 40 by resident. Psychopharmacology: None
Length of follow-up: 1 year, 3 months from consultation and still in psychotherapy.
Setting of follow-up: Videotaped interview in Brief Therapy Clinic with criteria for dynamic change defined in advance.

Input Variables

1. Orientation (focus): I posed to her that her vocal directness about her problem saturation drove people away and left her lonely. I also challenged her entitlement to a world that would be different. Could she attend to who could listen and who could not?
2. Topography of her dilemma (motivation and helping alliance): She was certainly motivated to talk in therapy about her misery, where it was indeed acceptable. Whether she could improve her eye in the world was the question. In retrospect, it is clear that this pole of distance in her near/far dilemma never came into focus for me. I imagine she felt very helpless and defaulted upon (basic fault; see Figure 15.5).
3. Available territory (systemic opportunities): Pretty alone in the world, with not much to show for her degree to come as an undergraduate.

Output Variables

Symptomatic change: Still depressed.
Dynamic change criteria

1. a. Less forcing of the world: Modest change. She is still unduly hopeful, and angry. She did tell her mother not to put her down. She did refuse to continue asking her friends to hear all her tribulations.
   b. Accepting and yielding: She has gotten a decent boss, and therapist, and two friends, and a little family support from sister and father.
2. Extravagance and vegetation in other domains: Similarly on the edge of re-entry into an intimacy. Forcing and yielding in other domains: She is in pretty much the same story in work, love, family, with the exceptions noted.
3. (Transcendence): Her gallows humor is very enjoyable and protects her from pain, but verges on cynicism. It is an attempt at a development on the shadow side.

DISCUSSION: This is a classic situation for young women who are idealists about the world. When this is held to strictly, it leads to bitterness. Certainly, it is worsened by lack of connections (her ecology). My intuitive response was to tell her about Solidarity in Poland as a movement with a program for thirty million souls like herself. This is the Polish dilemma. If you believe in authorities, you will be crushed. If you disbelieve and get mad, you will be discredited. The middle path is to appeal to those who actually care for you.

Availability of Territory

Case 7. Basilar Artery Migraine

Patient's age: 20. Sex: Female. Marital status: Single. Occupation: Student. Sessions: 10 in 4 months by resident, after 3 hours by myself; 1 hour of preliminary evaluation and 2 hours of videotaped consultation in the clinic. Psychopharmacology: None
Length of follow-up: 2 years from initial consultation, 1 year and 8 months from end of psychotherapy.
Setting of follow-up: Videotaped interview in Brief Therapy Clinic with criteria for dynamic change specified in advance.

Input Variables

1. Orientation (focus): Trying to be wonderful, she ends up enraged with nowhere to go with it. See Chapter 7 for narrative.
2. Topography of her dilemma (motivation and helping alliance): If she is wonderfully agreeable, she gets pushed around. If she is assertive, she'll hurt somebody. There is tremendous expressive ability verbally and nonverbally, and self-delight in becoming known, and ability to face pain, and make difficult decisions. See Figure 7.3.
3. Available territory (systemic opportunities): Considerable support from her family to own her hatred, and considerable opportunity for her developing self-expression in the university.

Output Variables

Symptomatic Change: Florid, major distress on all categories of SCL-90, to virtually zero at follow-up. No recurrence of the "migraine" despite two Christmases and two summers at home (where they occurred).
Dynamic change criteria

1. a. Handling powerful women: Feeling less powerful, or too powerful. Marvelous change in no longer putting mother, grandmother, and sister on a pedestal, and no longer being driven to be the wonderful granddaughter, daughter, and sister.

   b. Being on her own, no longer the baby: Also impressive change in being a grown-up young woman, taking care of school. Of course, graduation from college will test this more deeply.
2. Learning I changes in other domains: The resolution of her pleasing/independence dilemma has generalized to roommates, boyfriend, school, and myself as interviewer. If she has residual tendencies to subserve men, she told me that Freud made too much of his own penis!
3. (Transcendence): There is remarkable poise here between fitting the world and fitting herself, which I would call the region of the equipoise or equanimity. The question is its stability under great forces, such as the slog of graduate school, the perversity of marriage, the hierarchy of career.

DISCUSSION: Another beautiful brief therapy with major dynamic change in terms of Learning I and II. Learning III cannot be judged without the major tests of adult life. A twenty-three-year-old can be pretty poised in the context of university, and slip badly in a harsh world of pulls to the right to fit it, and pulls to the left in outraged reaction. In other words, Anna Karenina is still in the late blue mist of childhood prolonged by college, and has yet to enter the narrow defile of adult life where the forces are huge to distort this achievement.

Case 8. A Good Girl Going to Heaven

Patient's age: 45. Sex: Female. Marital status: Married. Occupation: Clerk. Sessions: 85 in 5 years with three residents; two consultations by myself, one inpatient, one videotaped in Brief Therapy Clinic. Psychopharmacology: Several antidepressants
Length of follow-up: 1 year and 3 months from my first consultation on inpatient service; patient still in therapy with the resident.
Setting of follow-up: Videotaped interview in Brief Therapy Clinic with criteria for dynamic change specified in advance.

Input Variables

1. Orientation (focus): Her subservience is taken advantage of, quite like Thelma and Louise, while her rebellion is self-destructive in its sexual excitement, also quite like Thelma and Louise.
2. Topography of her dilemma (motivation and helping alliance): She is dead blank in her servitude, and as engaging as Italian opera in her dancing, which is out of control. As one of the residents observing this discussion said: Good girls go to heaven/Bad girls go everywhere. Unfortunately, both are myths (see Figure 15.6).
3. Available territory (systemic opportunities): Very poor—her husband and her son make scandalous use of her. She has no allies in the world, except

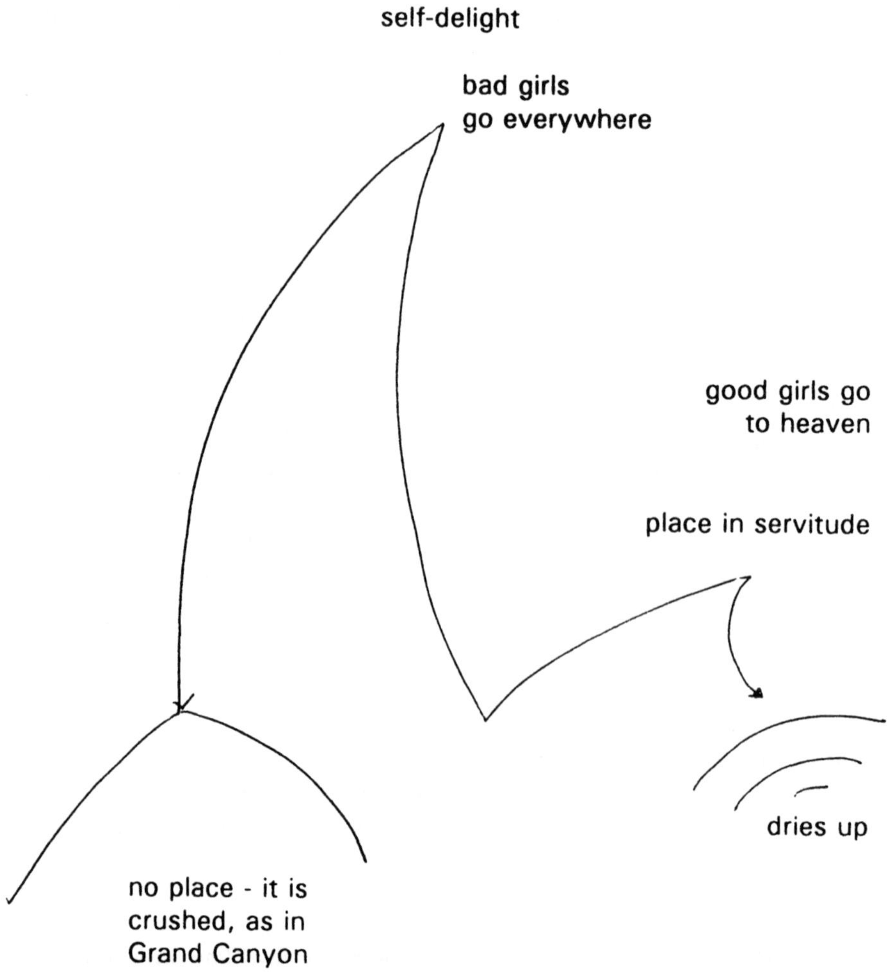

Figure 15.6. Good and bad girls.

working for her sister as a clerk, which she is proud of. Her work ethic engages here, and keeps her head up.

Output Variables

Symptomatic change: Still immobilized in depression.

Dynamic Change Criteria

1. Assimilation of vigor is self-defeating and drives her back into infinite servitude: essentially, back to being ill-used by son and by husband.
2. Learning I in other dimensions: There aren't any.
3. (Transcendence): The humor is there, but it is wan in the face of her thin possibilities.

DISCUSSION: Here is the usual tragedy of women, not only in America (Gilligan, 1990), but in Africa (Ba, 1980), or in Europe (Selvini-Palazzoli et al., 1978): She has a place in servitude, and she has no place in her beautiful self-expression, such as in her dancing. Without considerable backing, from family and from a profession, she is going to go down. A little therapy, with correct orientation and some longing to be understood, finds her beautifully, but the currents drown her in their ferocity. She is no match for these forces on her own in a harsh world, like Jane Roe of *Roe vs. Wade* (McCorvey, 1994).

Case 9. Being Fully at Home in Baseball

Patient's age: 21. Sex: M. Marital status: S. Work: Student. Sessions: Two series of 12 sessions each in 4 months with two different residents; 2 consultations with me videotaped in Brief Therapy Clinic; 27 hours in all over 3 years. Psychopharmacology: Imipramine, 50 mg, discontinued during brief therapy.
Length of follow-up: 3 years and 3 months from original consultation; still in therapy with second resident at that time.
Setting of follow-up: Videotaped consultation in Brief Therapy Clinic.

Input Variables

1. Orientation (focus): See Chapter 8 for narrative. I take him to what he deeply resents, being subjected to tests, because it cannot be avoided in the world.
2. Topography of his dilemma (motivation and helping alliance): If he is put into a roller coaster and sent for a ride, he hates it. If he is free as in baseball, he is perfectly natural. However beautiful the shadow story, he has to return to the world. There he is full of hatred at these intrusions. Then he is likely to delay and obfuscate. See Figure 8.2.
3. Available territory (systemic opportunities): Marvelous use of umpiring as middle ground. He is really on his own from an impoverished family.

Output Variables

Symptomatic change: Formal data not available, but his second resident's termination note suggests that panic attacks were successfully treated by him with Imipramine.
Dynamic change criteria

1. Delaying operations, with panic (versus facing his tests, and bearing his anger): Some good signs, like writing ex-girlfriend and keeping journal, of clarity. Also bought himself a quality mountain bike. Yet in therapy itself, he was often obscure in a cloud of ambiguity and distance.
2. Learning I in other dimensions: Visually, he is completely different. First met, he looked like a marginal Vietnam Vet in khakis, while now he is a handsome man who looks acceptable.
3. (Transcendence): This man has a great deal of profundity of self-expression.

DISCUSSION: Like the "Children of the Garden Island" (Werner, 1989) with determination, this man goes forward with ever so little backing. Beautifully free like Huck he thrives, but going on land he is hurt and angry at its narrow tricks. Still, the challenge is to handle these tricks, which arouse tremendous hatred. From this he tends to run into obscurity. We will need time to see if he comes through. Most turn into woodchucks (see the woodchuck of Chapter 13).

Case 10. A Dog in Hell

Patient's age: 31. Sex: Male. Marital status: Single. Occupation: Student. Sessions: 172 by myself over 10 years. Psychopharmacology: None
Length of follow-up: 8 years. Setting of follow-up: Private consultation.

Input Variables

1. Orientation (focus): Secret stubbornness to prove himself, despite history as dog in hell.
2. Topography of his dilemma (motivation and helping alliance): His determination gets him through college, but then is misplaced in other domains in impossible battles for a job and for girlfriend (see Figure 15.7 and narrative in Chapter 1).

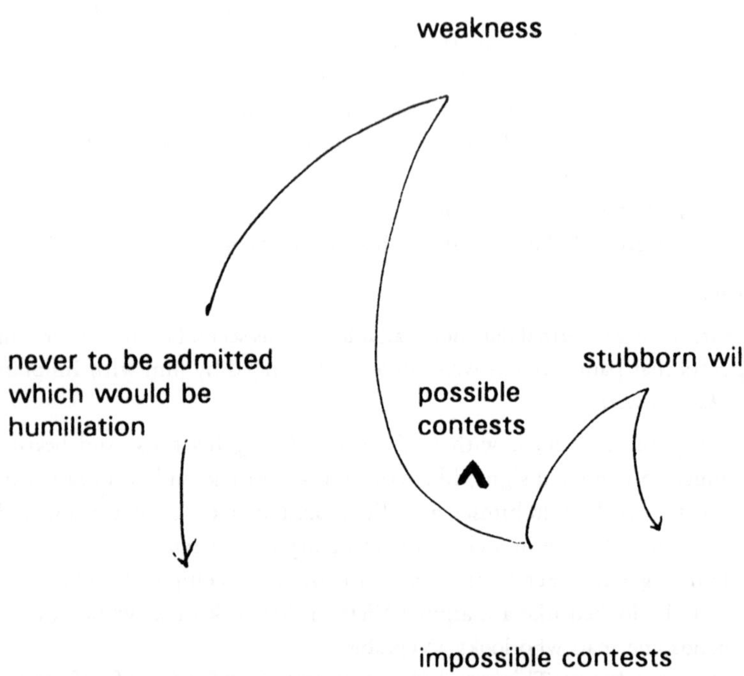

Figure 15.7. Dog in hell.

3. Available territory (systemic opportunities): Basically, he can fall back into his family like Biff of Miller's *Death of a Salesman,* but his father's ideas about success are no better than Willy Loman's.

Output Variables

Symptomatic change: No formal data; I find him recurrently depressed, yet more revivable in humor than his grim self I first knew.

Dynamic change criteria

1. Determination is only a good thing when it is applied to battles that can be won: He has spent the last five years after college in impossible battles to get a job and to get a girl when he has zero economics to offer.
2. Learning I in other domains: There are no other domains.
3. (Transcendence): There is humor, like that of Gogol, but it is vain without victories in battles that are possible.

DISCUSSION: This stubborn man may yet learn from his last five years of impossible battles to pick possible ones. He had a possible battle to finish college, and then got himself two impossible battles to get a job he couldn't qualify for and a woman he couldn't qualify for. Some people only learn by dire experience, and some don't. It is much harder without family backing, and connections, and sense, as Arthur Miller shows with Biff and Hap, Mr. Outside and Mr. Inside, both ruined.

Summary of Results

I would like to conclude this book with a summary of my ideas of research on brief psychotherapy and a summary of my findings in these cases. Essentially, I am arguing that a model that gets near to the complex drama of psychotherapy has to be a hierarchical theory. My model is that the psychotherapy has to be oriented to what the patient is overlooking that is ruining him, it has to engage sufficient motivation in the patient to do something else, and it has to find a territory in which that something else can be played to advantage. The results of the ten cases are summarized in Table 1. In broad summary, Cases 5, 6, and 8 went nowhere, while Case 10 had a significant success and came to a dead halt. All four of these cases are basically faulted in the benign sense. All four patients were attached to mythical ideas that collapsed in the territory of the outer world that had few resources for them. All four could not shift orientation to an alternative myth, for they would be dropped back into the faulted childhood. Thus, they lacked motivation for anything else. They doggedly stuck to something that would not work. So they faltered in a complex interaction of a dogged misorientation, a lack of motivation for the alternative or shadow myth, and a lack of territory that would be kind to their dogged project (see Figure 15.8).

In contrast, Cases 3, 4, and 7 are marvelous shifts that show the power of an accurate reorientation, motivation to undergo a shift into a shadow power, and

Table 1. Summary of Ten Cases of Brief Psychotherapy

Case	Learning I	Learning II	Learning III
1. A Vampire	+		
2. The Mythical Dimensions of J. Crew	+		
3. The French Bullet Train	+	+	±
4. Hamlet	+	+	±
5. The Grand Bartender	−		
6. Direct Young Woman (Polish dilemma)	−		
7. Basilar Artery Migraine	+	+	±
8. A Good Girl Going to Heaven	−		
9. Being Fully at Home in Baseball	+		
10. A Dog in Hell	±		

territory to play it out. Cases 1 and 2 show marvelous jumps from a reorientation in a single dream in highly motivated patients with available territory to work on. Case 9 also made a significant jump, but the outcome is in doubt because of his difficulty bearing anger or hatred of a limiting world without becoming cloudy. In this sense, the problem is quantitative, that is, whether or not he has adequate capacity to bear the strength of feeling that must be borne in a harsh world. He has an inner grasp of himself, but it has to be taken into the outer world.

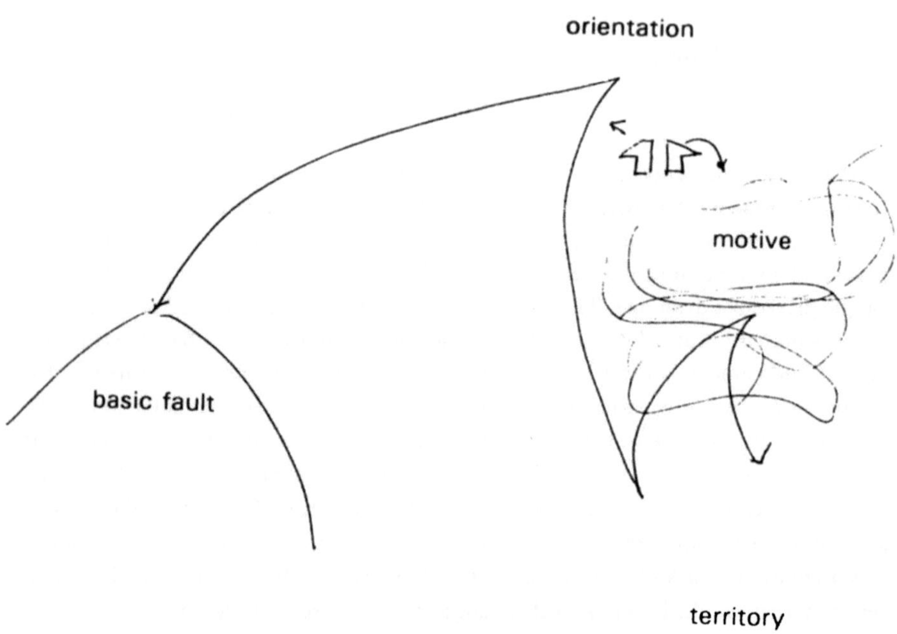

Figure 15.8. Doggedness.

References

Adams, H. (1961). *The education of Henry Adams.* Boston: Houghton Mifflin. (Original work published 1907)

Adams, H. (1986). *Mont Saint-Michel and Chartres.* New York: Penguin. (Original work published 1904)

Alexander, F., & French, T. M. (1946). *Psychoanalytic therapy, principles and applications.* New York: Ronald Press.

Allen, T. F. H., & Starr, T. B. (1982). *Hierarchy, perspectives for ecological complexity.* Chicago: University of Chicago Press.

Arendt, H. (1963). *Eichmann in Jerusalem. A report on the banality of evil.* New York: Penguin.

Asch, S. S. (1976). Varieties of negative therapeutic reaction and problems of technique. *Journal of the American Psychoanalytic Association, 24,* 383–407.

Ba, M. (1980). *So long a letter.* Portsmouth, NH: Heinemann.

Balint, M. (1952). New beginning and paranoid and depressive syndromes. *International Journal of Psychoanalysis, 33,* 214. (Reprinted in M. Balint, *Primary love and psychoanalytic technique.* New York: Liveright, 1953).

Balint, M. (1968). *The basic fault, therapeutic aspects of regression.* London: Tavistock.

Balint, E., & Norell, J. S. (1973). *Six minutes for the patient.* London: Tavistock.

Balint, M., Ornstein, P., & Ornstein, O. (1972). *Focal psychotherapy, an example of applied psychoanalysis.* London: Tavistock.

Balzac, H. de (1946). *Pere Goriot.* New York: The Modern Library. (Original work published 1835)

Bartsch, D. A., et al. (1990). Screening CMHC outpatients for physical illness. *Hospital and Community Psychiatry, 41,* 786.

Bateson, G. (1971). The cybernetics of "self": A theory of alcoholism. *Psychiatry, 34,* 1–17.

Bateson, G. (1972). *Steps toward an ecology of mind.* New York: Ballantine.

Bateson, G. (1979). *Mind and nature. A necessary unity.* New York: Bantam.

Beels, C. (1991). An interview with Chris Beels. Interviewed by S. Madigan. *Dulwich Centre Newsletter,* no. 4, pp. 13–21.

Bennett, H. J. (1993). *The New England Kernel of Medicine.*

Bennett M. J. (1983). Focal psychotherapy—terminable and interminable. *American Journal of Psychotherapy, 37,* 365–375.

Bennett, M. J. (1985). Focal behavioral psychotherapy for acute narcissistic injury: "De Mopes"—report of a case. *American Journal of Psychotherapy, 39,* 126–133.

Bernstein, B. (1973). *Class, codes and control.* St. Albin, Herts: Paladin.

Bibring, E. (1953). The mechanism of depression. In P. Greenacre (Ed.), *Affective disorders, Psychoanalytic contributions to their study.* New York: International Universities Press.

Bly, C. (1981). *Letters from the country.* New York: Harper & Row.

Bourdieu, P. (1977). *Outline of a theory of practice.* Translated by Richard Nice. Cambridge, England: Cambridge University Press.

Bourdieu, P. (1984). *Distinction: A social critique of the judgment of taste.* Translated by Richard Nice. Cambridge: Harvard University Press.

Bourdieu, P. (1988). *Homo academicus.* Translated by Peter Collier. Stanford, CA: Stanford University Press.

Brenman, M. (1952). On teasing and being teased: And the problem of "moral masochism". In *The psychoanalytic study of the child, VII* (pp. 264–285).

Breuer, J., & Freud, S. (1966). *Studies on hysteria.* New York: Avon Press. (Original work published 1895)

Brodsky, J. (1986). *Less than one. Selected essays.* New York: Farrar, Straus & Giroux.

Brodsky, J. (1988). Uncommon visage. The Nobel lecture. *The New Republic,* January 4 and 11.

Callahan, J., & Sashin, J. I. (1990). Predictive models in psychoanalysis. *Behavioral Science, 35,* 60–76.

Calvino, I. (1972). *Invisible cities.* Translated from Italian by William Weaver. New York: Harcourt Brace Jovanovich.

Campbell, J. (1949). *The hero with a thousand faces.* Princeton, NJ: Princeton University Press.

Campbell, J. (1964). *The masks of God: Occidental mythology.* New York: Penguin.

Canetti, E. (1981). *Crowds and power.* Translated from the German by Carol Stewart. New York: Continuum. (Original work published 1960).

Charbonnier, G. (1969). *Conversations with Claude Levi-Strauss.* Translated by John and Doreen Weightman. London: Jonathan Cape.

Colinvaux, P. (1983). Human history: A consequence of plastic niche but fixed breeding strategy. In J. B. Calhoun (Ed.), *Environment and population.* New York: Praeger.

Davanloo, H. (1986). Intensive short-term psychotherapy with highly resistant patients. I. Handling resistance. *International Journal of Short-Term Psychotherapy, 1,* 107–133.

De Shazer, S. (1987). Minimal elegance. *Family Therapy Networker,* October, pp. 57–60.

De St. Exupery, A. (1939). *Wind, sand, and stars.* Translated by Lewis Galantiere. New York: Harcourt Brace Jovanovich.

Dickinson, E. (1858–1865). *The complete poems of Emily Dickinson.* T. H. Johnson (Ed.). Boston: Little Brown.

Doyle, A. C. (1929). *Sherlock Holmes. The complete long stories.* London: John Murray.

Edelman, G. M. (1979). Group selection and phasic reentrant signaling: A theory of higher brain function. In G. M. Edelman & V. B. Mountcastle (Eds.), *The mindful brain* (pp. 51–100). Cambridge, MA: MIT Press.

Edelman, G. M. (1982). Through a computer darkly: Group selection and higher brain function. *Bulletin of the American Academy of Arts and Sciences, 36,* 20–49.

Edelman, G. M. (1985). Neural Darwinism: Population thinking and higher brain function. In M. Shafto (Ed.), *How we know* (pp. 1–30). San Francisco: Harper & Row.

Edelman, G. M. (1989). *Topobiology. An introduction to molecular biology.* New York: Basic Books.

Eliot, G. (1965). *Middlemarch.* Harmondworth, Middlesex, England: Penguin. (Original work published 1871)

El Saadawi, N. (1983). *Woman at point zero.* Translated by Sherif Hetata. London: Zed Books. (Original work published 1975)

Erikson, E. H. (1954). The dream specimen of psychoanalysis. *Journal of the American Psychoanalytical Association, 2,* 5–56.

Flaubert, G. (1857). *Madame Bovary.* Translated by Paul de Man. New York: Norton, 1965.

Forster, E. M. (1924). *Passage to India.* New York: Harcourt, Brace and World.

Forster, E. M. (1941). *Howard's end.* Harmondsworth, Middlesex, England: Penguin Books.

Foucault, M. (1975). *Discipline and punish. The birth of the prison.* Translated from the French by Alan Sheridan. New York: Vintage, 1979.

Foucault, M. (1980). In C. Gordon (Eds.), *Power/knowledge. Selected interviews and other writings.* New York: Pantheon.

Freire, P. (1970). *Pedagogy of the oppressed.* New York: Herder and Herder.

Freud, S. (1965). *The interpretation of dreams.* New York: Avon. (Original work published 1900).

Freud, S. (1975). Notes upon a case of obsessional neurosis. In J. Strachey (Ed. and Trans.), *The standard edition of the complete psychological works of Sigmund Freud* (Vol. 10, pp. 153–318). New York: Norton. (Original work published 1909)

Freud, S. (1963a). Recommendations for physicians on the psychoanalytic method of treatment. In P. Rieff (Ed.), *Freud, therapy and technique* New York: Collier. (Original work published 1912, 1913, 1914, 1915)

Freud, S. (1915–1917). *Introductory lectures to psychoanalysis.* Published in English as *A general introduction to psychoanalysis.* New York: Pocket Books, 1953.

Freud, S. (1963b). Mourning and melancholia. In P. Rieff (Ed.), *General psychological theory, papers on meta-psychology.* New York: Collier. (Original work published 1917)

Freud, S. (1975). From the history of an infantile neurosis. In J. Strachey (Ed. and Trans.), The *Standard edition of the complete psychological works of Sigmund Freud* (Vol. 17). New York: Norton. (Original work published 1918)

Fussell, P. (1983). *Class.* New York: Ballantine.

Galdston, I. (1954). Sophocles contra Freud: A reassessment of the Oedipus Complex. *Bulletin New York Academy Medicine, 30,* 803–817.

Gardner, H. (1971). *Religion and literature.* London: Faber and Faber.

Gardner, M. (1971). *The wolf man by the wolf man.* New York: Basic Books.

Gilligan, C. (1982). *In a different voice: Psychological theory and women's developments.* Cambridge, MA: Harvard University Press.

Gilligan, C. (1990). Joining the resistance: Psychology, politics, girls and women. *Michigan Quarterly Review,* XXIX *4,* 501–536.

Goethe, J. W. V. (1832). *Faust.* Translated by L. MacNeice. New York: Oxford, University Press, 1951.

Gogol, N. (1835). Nevsky Prospect. In L. J. Kent (Eds.), *The complete tales of Nikolai Gogol.* Volume I (pp. 207–238). Chicago: University of Chicago Press, 1985.

Gogol, N. (1836). The nose. In L. J. Kent (Eds.), *The complete tales of Nikolai Gogol.* Volume II (pp. 215–239). Chicago: University of Chicago Press, 1985.

Grimm, J. L. K. (1819). *Grimm's tales for young and old.* Translated by R. Mannheim. New York: Doubleday, 1977.

Guntrip, H. (1968). *Schizoid phenomena, object-relations and the self.* New York: International Universities Press.

Gustafson, J. P. (1976). The group matrix of individual therapy with Plains Indian people. *Contemporary Psychoanalysis, 12,* 227–239.

Gustafson, J. P. (1984). An integration of brief psychotherapy. *American Journal of Psychiatry, 141,* 935–944.

Gustafson, J. P. (1986). *The complex secret of brief psychotherapy.* New York: Norton. Reissued in paperback, 1995, Jason Aronson, New York.

Gustafson, J. P. (1987). The neighboring field of brief individual psychotherapy. *Journal of Marital and Family Therapy, 13,* 409–422.

Gustafson, J. P. (1989, July). A scientific journey of twenty years. *Journal of Strategic and Systemic Therapies.*

Gustafson, J. P. (1990). The great simplifying conventions of brief psychotherapy. In J. K. Zeig & S. G. Gilligan (Eds.), *Brief therapy, myths, methods and metaphors.* New York: Brunner/Mazel.

Gustafson, J. P. (1992). *Self-delight in a harsh world. The main stories of individual, marital and family psychotherapy.* New York: Norton.

Gustafson, J. P. (in press). The ecology of OCD. In J. Greist and J. Jefferson (Eds.), *OCD.* Washington: American Psychiatric Press.

Gustafson, J. P. (1967). Hallucinoia, the release of phantoms in schizophrenia. Unpublished doctoral dissertation, Harvard Medical School.

Gustafson, J. P. (unpublished a). Freud's unsolved problems.

Gustafson, J. P. (unpublished b). Finding and going forward: The two great challenges of long-term psychotherapy.

Gustafson, J. P. (1995). *Brief Versus Long Psychotherapy in Practice.* New York: Jason Aronson.

Gustafson, J. P., & Cooper, L. W. (1990). *The modern contest, a systemic guide to the pattern that connects individual psychotherapy, family therapy, group work, teaching, organizational life, and large-scale social problems.* New York: Norton.

Haley, J. (1966). Toward a theory of pathological systems. In G. N. Zuk & I. Boszormenyi-Nagy (Eds.), *Family therapy and disturbed families.* Palo Alto: Science and Behavior Books.

Hall, R. C. W., Beresford, T. P., & Popkin, M. K. (1982). The medical care of psychiatric patients. *Hospital and Community Psychiatry, 33,* 25.

Hall, R. C. W., et al. (1978). Physical illness presenting as psychiatric disease. *Archives of General Psychiatry, 35,* 1315.

Hardy, T. (1878). *The return of the native.* New York: Penguin, 1978.

Hardy, T. (1886). *The mayor of Casterbridge.* New York: Pocket Books, 1956.

Havens, L. (1965). The anatomy of a suicide. *New England Journal of Medicine, 272,* 401–406.

Hesse, H. (1970). *Magister Ludi (the glass bead game).* R. Winston & C. Winston (Trans.). New York: Bantam. (Original work published 1970)

Hoffman, L. (1975). Enmeshment and the too richly cross-joined system. *Family Process 14,* 457–469.

Jacobson, E. (1953). Contribution to the metapsychology of cyclothymic depression. In P. Greenacre (Ed.), *Affective disorders, psychoanalytic contributions to their study.* New York: International Universities Press.

James, W. (1958). *The varieties of religious experience.* New York: Mentor. (Original work published 1902)

Jerome, St. (4th century A.D.). *Saint Jerome lettres.* Translated by Jerome Labourt. Paris: Societe D'Edition Les Belles Lettres, 1953.

Jones, E. (1923). The God complex. The belief that one is God, and the resulting character traits. In E. Jones (Ed.), *Essays in applied psychoanalysis.* London: International Psychoanalytic Press.

Joyce, J. (1914). *Ulysses.* New York: Modern Library, 1961.

Jung, C. G. (1972). The relations between the ego and the unconscious. In J. Campbell (Ed.), *The portable Jung.* New York: Penguin. (Original work published in 1916)

Jung, C. G. (1971). Marriage as a psychological relationship. In J. Campbell (Eds.), *The portable Jung.* New York: Penguin. (Original work published, 1925)

Jung, C. G. (1933). Dream-analysis in its practical application. In C. G. Jung (Eds.), *Modern man in search of a soul.* Translated by W. S. Dell and Cary F. Baynes. New York: Harcourt, Brace.

Jung, C. G. (1985). *The practice of psychotherapy.* Princeton, NJ: Princeton University Press. (Original work published 1954)

Jung, C. G. (1989). *Memories, dreams and reflections.* Recorded and edited by A. Jaffe. Translated from the German by R. and C. Winston. New York: Vintage Books. (Original work published 1962)

Kaku, M. (1994). *Hyperspace.* New York: Oxford University Press.

Kernberg, O., Selzer, M. A., Koenigsberg, H. W., Carr, A. C., & Appelbaum, A. H. (1988). *Psychodynamic psychotherapy of borderline patients.* New York: Basic Books.

Koch, K. (1973). *Rose, where did you get that red? Teaching great poetry to children.* New York: Vintage Books.

Koran, L. M., (1989). Medical evaluation of psychiatric patients. *Archives of General Psychiatry, 46,* 733.

Koranyi, E. K. (1979). Morbidity and ratio of undiagnosed physical illnesses in a psychiatric clinic population. *Archives of General Psychiatry, 36,* 414–419.

Korsch, B. M., & Negrete, V. F. (1972). Doctor-patient communication. *Scientific American, 227,* 66–74.

Kramer, P. (1993). Degrees of separation. *Psychiatric Times,* September, 1993.

Kuper, A., & Stone, A. A. (1982). The dream of Irma's injection: A structural analysis. *American Journal of Psychiatry, 139,* 1225–1234.

Lawrence, D. H. (1885–1930). *Birds, beasts and the third thing.* New York: Viking, 1982.

Lawrence, D. H. (1959). *Selected poems.* New York: Viking Press.

Lifton, R. J. (1986). *The Nazi doctors.* New York: Basic Books.

Luborsky, L., Crits-Cristoph, P., Mintz, J., & Auerbach, A. (1988). *Who will benefit from psychotherapy.* New York: Basic Books.

Main, T. F. (1957). The ailment. *British Journal of Medical Psychology, 30,* 129–145.

Malan, D. (1976a). *The frontier of brief psychotherapy.* New York: Plenum.

Malan, D. (1976b). *Toward the validation of dynamic psychotherapy.* New York: Plenum.

Malan, D. (1979). *Individual psychotherapy and the science of psychodynamics.* London: Butterworth.

Malan, D., Balfour, F. H. G., Hood, V. G., & Shooter, A. M. N. (1976). Group psychotherapy. A long-term follow-up study. *Archives of General Psychiatry, 33,* 1303–1315.

Malan, D. H., Health, E. S., Bacal, H. A., & Balfour, F. H. G. (1975). Psychodynamic changes in untreated neurotic patients. II. Apparently genuine improvements. *Archives of General Psychiatry, 32,* 110–126.

Mann, J. (1973). *Time-limited psychotherapy.* Cambridge, MA: Harvard University Press.

Margolick, D. (1993). Lisa's bright shining future is laid to rest at Arlington. *New York Times,* July 17, p. 1.

Margulies, A. (1989). *The empathic imagination.* New York: Norton.

Marks, I. (1987). *Fears, phobias, and rituals, the nature of anxiety and panic disorders.* New York: Oxford University Press.

Maturana, H. F., & Varela, F. J. (1980). *Autopoiesis and cognition. The realization of the living.* Boston: D. Reidel.

Mayman, M., & Faris, M. (1960). Early memories as expressions of relationship paradigms. *American Journal of Orthopsychiatry, 30,* 507–520.

McCorvey, N. (1994). *I am Roe: My life, Roe vs. Wade and freedom of choice.* New York: HarperCollins.

Merton, T. (1948). *The seven story mountain.* New York: Harcourt Brace Jovanovich.

Muecke, L. N., & Krueger, D. W. (1981). Physical findings in a psychiatric outpatient clinic. *American Journal of Psychiatry, 138,* 1241–1242.

Newton, P. (1979). *The accursed correspondence: The Freud/Jung letters.* University Publishing, Spring.

Orwell, G. (1946). The politics of the English language. In G. Orwell (Ed.), *A collection of essays by George Orwell.* New York: Harcourt Brace Jovanovich.

Poirier, R. (1966). *A world elsewhere. The place of style in American literature.* Madison, WI: University of Wisconsin Press.

Popper, K. R. (1965). *The logic of scientific discovery.* New York: Harper & Row. (Original work published 1934)

Reich, W. (1949). *Character analysis.* New York: Farrar, Straus, & Giroux. (Original work published 1933)

Rilke, R. M. (1938). *Translations from the poetry of Rainer Maria Rilke.* Translated by M. D. Herder Norton. New York: Norton.

Rose, P. (1984). *Parallel lives. Five Victorian marriages.* New York: Random House.

Ryle, A. (1990). *Cognitive-analytic therapy. A new integration in brief psychotherapy.* New York: Wiley.

Ryle, A. (1994). Introduction to cognitive-analytic therapy. *International Journal of Short-Term Psychotherapy* 9, 93–110.

Selvini-Palazzoli, M. (1980). Why a long interval between sessions. The therapist control of the family-therapist suprasystem. In M. Andolfi & I. Zwerling (Eds.), *Dimensions of family therapy.* New York: Guilford Press.

Selvini-Palazzoli, M. (1985). The problem of the sibling as referring person. *Journal of Marital and Family Therapy, 11,* 21–34.

Selvini-Palazolli, M., (1986). *The hidden games of organizations.* New York: Pantheon.

Selvini-Palazzoli, M., Boscolo, L., Cecchin, G. F., & Prata, G. (1977). Family rituals: A powerful tool in family therapy. *Family Process, 16,* 445–453.

Selvini-Palazzoli, M., Boscolo, L., Cecchin, G. F., & Prata, G. (1978). *Paradox and counter-paradox: A new model in the therapy of the family in schizophrenic transactions.* New York: Jason Aronson.

Selvini-Palazzoli, M., Cirillo, S., Selvini, M., & Sorrentino, A. M. (1989). *Family games, general models of psychotic process in the family.* New York: Norton.

Shapiro, D. (1976). The analyst's own analysis. *Journal of the American Psychoanalytic Association, 24,* 5.

Smith, G., & Tiggeman, J. (1989). Seeing teenagers separately: New stories in the family. *Dulwich Centre Newsletter,* Winter, 1989, pp. 3–9.

Sox, H. C., (1989). A medical algorithm for detecting disease in psychiatric patients. *Hospital and Community Psychiatry, 40,* 1270.

Strupp, H. H., & Binder, J. (1984). *Psychotherapy in a new key: Time-limited dynamic psychotherapy.* New York: Basic Books.

Sullivan, H. S. (1954). *The psychiatric interview.* New York: Norton.

Sullivan, H. S. (1956). *Clinical studies in psychiatry.* New York: Norton.

Terkel, S. (1972). *Working.* New York: Avon.

Thoreau, H. D. (1982). Walden. In *The portable Thoreau.* New York: Penguin. (Originally published 1859)

Tiggeman, J., & Smith, G. (1989). Adolescent 'shock therapy': Teenagers shocking their critics. *Dulwich Centre Newsletter,* Winter, pp. 10–16.

Tolstoy, L. *War and peace.* New York: Modern Library. (Original work published 1869)

Tolstoy, L. (1970). *Anna Karenina.* New York: Norton. (Original work published 1875)

Turner, A. K. (1993). *The history of hell.* New York: Harcourt, Brace.

Turquet, P. (1975). Threats to identity in the large group. In L. Kreeger (Ed.), *The large group, dynamics and therapy.* London: Constable.

Vosnesensky, A. (1966). *Antiworlds. Poetry by Andrei Vosnesensky.* Translated by Patricia Blake and Max Hayward. New York: Basic Books.

Weber, M. (1958). *The Protestant ethic and the spirit of capitalism.* Translated by Talcott Parsons. New York: Charles Scribner's Sons. (Original work published 1904–1905)

Weekley, E. (1967). *An etymological dictionary of modern English.* New York: Dover.

Weiden, P., & Havens, L. (1994). Psychotherapeutic management techniques in the treatment of outpatients with schizophrenia. *Hospital and Community Psychiatry, 45,* 549–555.

Weil, S. (1993). The Iliad, or the poem of force. Translated by Richard Ringler. In R. Ringler (Ed.), *Dilemmas of War and Peace: A Source Book.* London: Routledge. (Original work published 1937)

Weiss, J., & Sampson, H. (1986). *The psychoanalytic process.* New York: Guilford.

Wells, K. B., Golding, J. M., & Burnam, M. A. (1989). Chronic medical conditions in a sample of the general population with anxiety, affective and substance use disorders. *American Journal of Psychiatry, 146,* 1440.

Werner, E. E. (1989). Children of the Garden Island. *Scientific American,* April, pp. 106–111.

White, M. (1984). Marital therapy: Practical approaches to long-standing problems. *Australian and New Zealand Journal of Family Therapy, 5,* 27–43.

White, M. (1989). *Selected papers.* Adelaide, South Australia: Dulwich Centre Publications.

White, M., & Epston, D. (1990). *Narrative means to therapeutic ends.* New York: Norton.

Winnicott, D. W. (1971a). *Playing and reality.* London: Tavistock.

Winnicott, D. W. (1971b). *Therapeutic consultations in child psychiatry.* New York: Basic Books.

Bibliography

Agee, J. (1938). *A death in the family.* New York: Avon Books, 1959.

Alexander, F., & French, T. M. (1946). *Psychoanalytic therapy, principles and applications.* New York: Ronald Press.

Alighieri, D. (1314). *Inferno.* Translation by 20 contemporary poets, D. Halpern (Ed.) New York: Ecco, 1993.

Carroll, L. (1865). *Alice in Wonderland.* Illustrated by Michael Hague. New York: Henry Holt and Company, 1865.

Eliot, G. (1871). *Middlemarch.* Harmondworth, Middlesex, England: Penguin, 1965.

Flaubert, G. (1857). *Madame Bovary.* New York: Paul de Man (Trans.). Norton, 1965.

Forster, E. M. (1924). *Passage to India.* New York: Harcourt, Brace and World.

Forster, E. M. (1941). *Howard's end.* Harmondsworth, Middlesex, England: Penguin Books.

Goethe, J. W. V. (1832). *Faust.* Translated by L. MacNeice. New York: Oxford University Press, 1951.

Gogol, N. (1835). Nevsky Prospect. In L. J. Kent (Eds.), *The complete tales of Nikolai Gogol.* Volume I (pp. 207–238). Chicago: University of Chicago Press, 1985.

Gogol, N. (1836). The nose. In L. J. Kent (Eds.), *The complete tales of Nikolai Gogol.* Volume II (pp. 215–239). Chicago: University of Chicago Press, 1985.

Grimm, J. L. K. (1819). *Grimm's tales for young and old.* R. Mannheim (Trans.) New York: Doubleday, 1977.

Hardy, T. (1878). *The return of the native.* New York: Penguin, 1978.

Hardy, T. (1886). *The mayor of Casterbridge.* New York: Pocket Books, 1956.

Homer, (c. 850 B.C.). *The iliad.* Translated by Robert Fitzgerald. Garden City, NY: Anchor Books, 1974.

Homer (c. 850 B.C.) *The odyssey.* New York: Anchor Books, 1963. Robert Fitzgerald (Trans.).

Irving, W. (1829). *Rip Van Winkle, or the strange men of the mountains.* New York: Scholastic, Inc., 1975.

Hughes, T. (1991). *The essential Shakespeare.* New York: Ecco Press.

James, H. (1903). The beast in the jungle. In D. Grant (Eds.), *American short stories.* London: Oxford University Press, 1972.

Kafka, F. (1883–1924). The judgment. In (Eds.), *F. Kafka: The penal colony: Stories and short pieces.* W. and E. Muir (Trans.). New York: Schocken.

Kafka, F. (1883–1924). *Metamorphosis.* A. I. Lloyd (Trans.). New York:

Melville, H. (1851). *Moby-Dick or, The whale.* Boston: Houghton Mifflin, 1956.

Melville, H. (1853). Bartleby the scrivener. In R. V. Cassill (Eds.), *The Norton anthology of short fiction.* New York: Norton, 1986.

Miller, A. (1950). *Death of a salesman.* New York: Viking.

Nietzsche, F. (1844–1900). *The portable Nietzsche.* W. Kaufman (Ed.). New York: Viking, 1954.

Pascal (1662). *Pensees.* Translated with an introduction by A. J. Krailsheimer. London: Penguin, 1966.

Percy, W. (1975). Metaphor as mistake. In W. Percy (Eds.), *The message in the bottle.* New York: Farrar, Straus, & Giroux.

Plato (427–347 B.C.). *Symposium.* R. G. Bury (Ed.). Cambridge: W. Heffer, 1932.

Porter, K. (1935). Theft. In R. V. Cassill (Eds.), *The Norton anthology of short fiction.* New York: Norton, 1986.

Rostand, E. (1898). *Cyrano de Bergerac.* A. Gertrude Hall (Trans.). New York: Doubleday.

Shakespeare, W. (1600). The life of King Henry the Fifth. In *William Shakespeare: The complete works.* Alfred Harbage, General Editor. Baltimore, MD: Penguin Books, 1969, revised edition.

Shakespeare, W. (1600). Hamlet, Prince of Denmark. In *William Shakespeare: The complete works.* Alfred Harbage, General Editor. Baltimore, MD: Penguin Books, 1969, revised edition.

Shakespeare, W. (1604). Othello the Moor of Venice. In *William Shakespeare: The complete works.* Alfred Harbage, General Editor. Baltimore, MD: Penguin Books, 1969, revised edition.

Shakespeare, W. (1605–1606). King Lear. In *William Shakespeare: The complete works.* Alfred Harbage, General Editor. Baltimore, MD: Penguin Books, 1969, revised edition.

Shakespeare, W. (1607). Antony and Cleopatra. In *William Shakespeare: The complete works.* Alfred Harbage, General Editor. Penguin Books, 1969, revised edition.

Shakespeare, W. (1608). Coriolanus. In A. H. General Editor (Eds.), *William Shakespeare: The complete works.* Alfred Harbage, General Editor. Baltimore, MD: Penguin Books, 1969, revised edition.

Shakespeare, W. (1611). The tempest. In *William Shakespeare: The complete works.* Alfred Harbage, General Editor. Baltimore, MD: Penguin Books, 1969, revised edition.

Sophocles (427–426 B.C.). Oedipus the king. D. Grene (Trans.). In D. Grove & R. Lattimore (Eds.), *Sophocles I: The complete Greek tragedies.* Chicago: University of Chicago Press, 1954.

Stevenson, R. L. (1886). *The strange case of Dr. Jekyll and Mr. Hyde.* New York: Puffin Books, 1985.

Thoreau, H. D. (1859). Walden. In *The portable Thoreau.* New York: Penguin, 1982.

Thurber (1942). The secret life of Walter Mitty. In R. V. Cassill (Eds.), *The Norton anthology of short fiction.* New York: Norton, 1986.

Twain, M. (1885). *The adventures of Huckleberry Finn.* New York: Collier, 1962.

Voltaire (1759). Candide. In B. R. Redman (Eds.), *The portable Voltaire.* New York: Viking Press, 1949.

Williams, W. C. (1950). The use of force. In R. V. Cassill (Eds.), *The Norton anthology of short fiction.* New York: Norton.

Woolf, V. (1927). *To the lighthouse.* New York: Harcourt Brace Jovanovich, 1981.

Index

MIX
Paper from responsible sources
FSC® C090958

If you have any concerns about our products
you can contact us on
ProductSafety@springernature.com

In case Publisher is established outside the EU,
the EU authorized representative is:
Springer Nature Customer Service Center GmbH
Europaplatz 3, 69115 Heidelberg, Germany

Printed by Libri Plureos GmbH
in Hamburg, Germany

MIX
Papier aus verantwortungsvollen Quellen
Paper from responsible sources
FSC® C105338

If you have any concerns about our products,
you can contact us on
ProductSafety@springernature.com

In case Publisher is established outside the EU,
the EU authorized representative is:
Springer Nature Customer Service Center GmbH
Europaplatz 3, 69115 Heidelberg, Germany

Printed by Libri Plureos GmbH
in Hamburg, Germany